# EveryWoman's®

## GUIDE TO

# *Healthier Eating*

# EveryWoman's®
## GUIDE TO
# *Healthier Eating*

### COMPILED AND EDITED BY
## Carol Tiffany

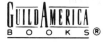

Doubleday Book & Music Clubs, Inc.
Garden City, New York

# Contents

# Introduction

*H*ere, at last, is a compact compendium of everything you need to know about diet and nutrition. In this easy-to-use guide, you'll find all the facts at your fingertips on how to

- Eat Slim/Keep Trim
- Count Your Calories/Count Your Fats
  (or Cholesterol or Sodium)
- Chart Your Way to Total Nutrition

So you want to be healthy/healthier? Looking good, feeling just right? With the help of this comprehensive collection of nutritional tools, you can make *today* Day One of a healthier, happier, more natural self.

Are you always trying to lose "just five more pounds"? Don't despair. Eating right and eating *light* can be enjoyable if you know how to eat well, if you know what you are eating and why.

*The New Doubleday Cookbook,* extensively researched and written by Jean Anderson and Elaine Hanna, supplies a host of healthful recipes—simple and delicious recipes with just a bit of a difference, whether it be an appetizer spread made out of eggplant, a pâté made with white kidney beans, or an apple soup.

You'll also find a week's menus for a low-calorie/low-fat diet, each menu delightfully varied and perfectly balanced, as well as interesting background material on the USDA's Food Guide Pyramid and on all the essential nutrients.

Perhaps you are more concerned with counting cholesterol (or sodium) than counting calories and fats. The *Food Counter* from the American Heart Association gives information on all of them in its extensive listing of foods.

Have you discovered that the only way you can maintain your weight is by expending extra calories through exercise? The *Calorie Counter/Calories Burned Per Hour* is a unique table that will show you just how many calories are used up during an hour's worth of over 30 daily activities and sports. At 1,222 calories burned per hour for a 125-pound woman, don't you think you might want to start running in place (at the rate of 140 counts a minute)? If that's too strenuous, there's always square dancing or tennis at around 350 calories per hour (while eating and sleeping are only 60 to 70 calories per hour). Take your pick; there's no excuse now that you know the facts.

What should you weigh, ideally? How many calories should you consume to maintain that weight? How much fat? What exactly is **in** that tasty turnip, that sinful sundae? Just turn to the appropriate chart or counter. Everything is here in this handy, quick-reference book, a complete guide to healthier eating that you'll find indispensable.

Look forward to looking good, feeling good—by eating right.

CAROL TIFFANY

# Eat Well/Keep Well

## FOOD GUIDE PYRAMID

*R*ecently the United States Department of Agriculture introduced the Food Guide Pyramid (see p. 4) to illustrate their dietary guidelines. Five basic food groups are shown in the three lower sections of the pyramid. The small tip at the top of the pyramid doesn't really count—it shows foods that should only be consumed sparingly.

The base of the Food Guide Pyramid shows the base of good eating, foods derived from grains: breads, cereals, rice, and pasta. They provide complex carbohydrates (starches), an important source of energy, especially in low-fat diets. They also provide vitamins, minerals, and fiber. *Recommended Daily Amounts:* 6 to 11 servings. Any of the following counts as 1 serving: 1 slice bread; 1 ounce ready-to-eat cereal; ½ cup cooked cereal, rice, or pasta.

The middle level shows foods that come from plants: vegetables and fruits. They are needed for the vitamins, minerals, and fiber they supply, and they are low in fat. *Recommended Daily Amounts:* 3 to 5 servings of vegetables; 2 to 4 servings of fruit. Any of the following counts as 1 serving: 1 cup raw leafy vegetables; ½ cup other vegetables, cooked or chopped raw; ¾ cup vegetable juice; 1 medium apple, ba-

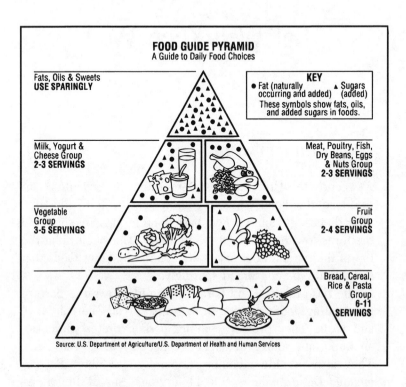

# FOOD GUIDE PYRAMID
A Guide to Daily Food Choices

Fats, Oils & Sweets
**USE SPARINGLY**

KEY
● Fat (naturally   ▲ Sugars
occurring and added)   (added)
These symbols show fats, oils,
and added sugars in foods.

Milk, Yogurt &
Cheese Group
**2-3 SERVINGS**

Meat, Poultry, Fish,
Dry Beans, Eggs
& Nuts Group
**2-3 SERVINGS**

Vegetable
Group
**3-5 SERVINGS**

Fruit
Group
**2-4 SERVINGS**

Bread, Cereal,
Rice & Pasta
Group
**6-11
SERVINGS**

Source: U.S. Department of Agriculture/U.S. Department of Health and Human Services

nana, or orange; ½ cup chopped, cooked, or canned fruit; ¾ cup fruit juice.

The top level of the pyramid shows two groups of foods that come mostly from animals: milk, yogurt, and cheese; and meat, poultry, fish, dry beans, eggs, and nuts. These foods are important for protein, vitamins, calcium, iron, and zinc. *Recommended Daily Amounts:* 2 to 3 servings of milk, yogurt, and cheese (this group is the best source of calcium); 2 to 3 servings of meat, poultry, fish, dry beans, eggs, and nuts. Any of the following counts as 1 serving: 1 cup milk or yogurt; 1½ ounces natural cheese; 2 ounces process cheese; 2 to 3 ounces cooked lean meat, poultry, or fish. *Note:* the total amount of servings in this second group should be the equivalent of 5 to 7 ounces of cooked lean meat, poultry, or fish per day; ½ cup cooked dry beans, 1 egg, or 2 tablespoons peanut butter counts as 1 ounce of lean meat.

The small tip of the pyramid shows foods that should only be used sparingly: fats, oils, and sweets such as salad dressings, salad oils, cream, butter, margarine, sugars, soft drinks, candies, and sweet desserts. They provide calories and not much else.

## *INDIVIDUAL NUTRIENTS*

There are three kinds of food: carbohydrates, proteins, and fats. (Calories come from these three food groups plus alcohol.) In addition, water, fiber, vitamins, and minerals are all necessary for good health. Let's examine them:

*Carbohydrates* contain 4 calories per gram. They burn faster and more efficiently than proteins or fats and are our best source of energy.

Sources of simple carbohydrates: refined sugars, syrups, candies, jams, sweetened soft drinks; fruits and fruit juices.

In certain people, simple carbohydrates can produce sugar "highs" and "lows."

Sources of complex carbohydrates: grain products, vegetables, potatoes, leafy greens. These foods often contain some fat as well as protein and are full of vitamins, minerals, and fiber.

*Proteins* contain 4 calories per gram. While they don't provide energy as fast as carbohydrates, they provide the essential minerals and amino acids, the body's building materials, which are necessary for the growth, maintenance, and repair of living cells.

Sources of animal protein: seafood, poultry, meat, dairy products, eggs.

Sources of plant protein: dried beans and peas, tofu, unhomogenized peanut butter, whole grains, vegetables.

*Fats* contain 9 calories per gram, more than twice as many as carbohydrates or proteins. While a little fat is necessary, eating more than the body requires produces unwanted body fat. Fats are found in animal foods (saturated fats) and plant foods (polyunsaturated and monounsaturated fats).

Sources of saturated fats (solid or almost solid at room temperature): poultry; meat; egg yolks; butter and butterfat; cocoa butter; coconut, palm kernel, and palm oil. They should be strictly limited in any healthy diet because they raise blood cholesterol levels in many people, increasing the risk of heart disease.

Sources of polyunsaturated fats (liquid at room temperature): corn, cottonseed, safflower, soybean, and sunflower oil; some fish. When used in conjunction with a diet low in cholesterol and saturated fats, they tend to lower blood cholesterol levels; however, recent research indicates that polyunsaturated fats may lower the good cholesterol (HDL) along with the bad cholesterol (LDL).

Sources of monounsaturated fats (liquid at room temperature): canola, olive, and peanut oil. When consumed in place of saturated fats, they seem to lower the bad cholesterol without lowering the good.

Sources of hydrogenated fats (polyunsaturated and monounsaturated fats that have been processed from liquids into semisolids): margarine, solid vegetable shortening, homogenized peanut butter. They should be limited because they behave like saturated fats in the body; hydrogenated margarines with 2 grams or less of saturated fat per tablespoon are acceptable.

What about *cholesterol?* Fats and cholesterol are not the same thing. Cholesterol is a fatlike substance produced by the body and also present in all animal foods: meat, poultry, fish, milk and milk products, egg yolks. Organ meats and egg yolks are especially high in dietary cholesterol; plant foods never contain cholesterol.

There are two types of cholesterol found in the blood: LDL and HDL. LDL is called the bad cholesterol; it increases the risk of heart disease by contributing to the buildup of plaque inside the arteries. HDL is called the good cholesterol; it helps flush out cholesterol from the bloodstream.

A diet high in cholesterol and saturated fat should be avoided; some health authorities recommend limiting dietary cholesterol to less than 300 milligrams a day. The goal is to keep your blood cholesterol level below 200. Since the latest medical evidence indicates that levels below 160 may be linked to increased risks (from other than heart disease), the safest cholesterol level may well be between 160 and 199, rather than lower.

*Water* is vital to your health. It helps to regulate temperature, aid digestion, and carry off body wastes. Drink 6 to 8 glasses every day. Please note: Coffee and tea don't count!

*Alcohol* is **not** a nutrient; it contains 7 calories per gram and has no nutritional benefit. Drink it in moderation—no more than one drink a day (12 ounces of beer, 5 ounces of wine, or 1½ ounces of liquor).

*Fiber* is found only in plant foods. Most foods with dietary fiber contain a mixture of insoluble and soluble fiber.

Sources of insoluble fiber: vegetables (unpeeled), whole-wheat breads and cereals, wheat bran. Insoluble fiber is thought to reduce the risk of colon cancer and stimulate bowel function.

Sources of soluble fiber: certain fruits and vegetables, beans, barley, oat bran, oatmeal. Soluble fiber has been shown to lower blood cholesterol levels in diets that are low in saturated fat and dietary cholesterol.

*Vitamins* are essential to good health. With a well-balanced diet, supplements are not usually required. Fresh foods, raw or lightly cooked, are the best sources of vitamins. Although a good vegetarian diet will contain most of the necessary nutrients, vegetarians may want to take a supplement to make up for the vitamin $B_{12}$ and vitamin D found in animal foods.

*Minerals* are equally essential. Calcium and sodium are two of the minerals that are stored in the body in large amounts.

While it is important to consume foods rich in calcium for strong bones and teeth, calcium supplements can be overdone (sometimes contributing to the formation of kidney stones) and cannot make up for a diet that has been perennially low in calcium. Good sources of calcium are milk, cheese, yogurt, dried beans, nuts, salmon, sardines with bones, oysters, collard greens, kale, turnip greens. Interesting to note: There is slightly **more** calcium in skim milk than in whole milk.

Sodium is often present in the body in excessive amounts. While we shouldn't take in more than 3,000 milligrams of sodium a day (some health authorities say not more than 2,400 milligrams), 1 teaspoon of salt provides almost 2,000 milligrams of sodium. Go easy on salt and foods high in sodium (cured meats, luncheon meats, many cheeses, most canned soups and vegetables, and soy sauce); too much sodium can contribute to high blood pressure.

## *TIME TO FOCUS*

The most important objective in any healthful diet should be to consume a rich variety of foods for energy, protein, vitamins, minerals, fiber. Beyond that, focus on foods that are low in fat, especially saturated fat, and low in cholesterol. The USDA and the American Heart Association recommend that Americans limit fat in their diets to 30 percent of their total calories; some health experts suggest 20 percent. In addition, the USDA and the American Heart Association recommend limiting **saturated** fat to 10 percent of total calories.

It's easy to figure the maximum grams of fat you should consume in a day:

**1.** Figure your calorie allowance for your ideal weight (see chart, pp. 12–13).

**2.** Multiply by 0.30 to get the recommended calories from fat per day.

**3.** Divide calories from fat per day by 9 (each gram of fat has 9 calories) to get the recommended grams of fat per day.

Go through the same process, but multiply by 0.10, then divide by 9, to arrive at the maximum amount of saturated fat you should consume in a day.

## THE BOTTOM LINE

*Strictly limit:*
   Fats (especially saturated fat)
   Cholesterol (especially organ meats, egg yolks)
   Added sugars
   Salt and sodium
   Alcohol

*Eat in moderation:*
   Low-fat milk, yogurt, cheese
   Lean meat, skinless poultry, fish
   Nuts

*Go for:*
   Breads, cereals, rice, and pasta (without added fats or sugars)
   Dried beans
   Skim milk, nonfat yogurt
   Vegetables (without added fats)
   Fruits (without added sugar)

Eat Well/Keep Well . . . go for it!

# Height/Weight/Calorie Chart

*T*o thwart the necessity of ever having to go on a diet, consult the following chart which shows desirable weights, based on height and frame size, and calorie needs, based on activity level. It will help you determine at a glance what you should weigh and how to maintain that desired weight:

# ADULT FEMALES

## *Calorie Level Based on Physical Activity*

| Height Without Shoes* | Frame Size | Desirable Weight** | Very Light (Calories) | Light (Calories) | Moderate (Calories) | Heavy (Calories) |
|---|---|---|---|---|---|---|
| 5'0" | Small | 106 (102–110) | 1,400 | 1,600 | 1,800 | 2,100 |
| | Medium | 113 (107–119) | 1,450 | 1,700 | 1,900 | 2,250 |
| | Large | 123 (115–131) | 1,600 | 1,850 | 2,100 | 2,450 |
| 5'1" | Small | 109 (105–113) | 1,400 | 1,650 | 1,850 | 2,200 |
| | Medium | 116 (110–122) | 1,500 | 1,750 | 1,950 | 2,300 |
| | Large | 126 (118–134) | 1,650 | 1,900 | 2,150 | 2,500 |
| 5'2" | Small | 112 (108–116) | 1,450 | 1,700 | 1,900 | 2,250 |
| | Medium | 119 (113–126) | 1,550 | 1,800 | 2,000 | 2,400 |
| | Large | 129 (121–138) | 1,700 | 1,950 | 2,200 | 2,600 |
| 5'3" | Small | 115 (111–119) | 1,500 | 1,750 | 1,950 | 2,300 |
| | Medium | 123 (116–130) | 1,600 | 1,850 | 2,100 | 2,450 |
| | Large | 133 (125–142) | 1,750 | 2,000 | 2,250 | 2,650 |
| 5'4" | Small | 118 (114–123) | 1,550 | 1,750 | 2,000 | 2,350 |
| | Medium | 127 (120–135) | 1,650 | 1,900 | 2,150 | 2,550 |
| | Large | 137 (129–146) | 1,800 | 2,050 | 2,350 | 2,750 |
| 5'5" | Small | 122 (118–127) | 1,600 | 1,850 | 2,050 | 2,450 |
| | Medium | 131 (124–139) | 1,700 | 1,950 | 2,250 | 2,600 |
| | Large | 141 (133–150) | 1,850 | 2,100 | 2,400 | 2,800 |

# ADULT FEMALES

## Calorie Level Based on Physical Activity

| Height Without Shoes* | Frame Size | Desirable Weight** | Very Light (Calories) | Light (Calories) | Moderate (Calories) | Heavy (Calories) |
|---|---|---|---|---|---|---|
| 5'6" | Small | 126 (122–131) | 1,650 | 1,900 | 2,150 | 2,500 |
| | Medium | 135 (128–143) | 1,750 | 2,050 | 2,300 | 2,700 |
| | Large | 145 (137–154) | 1,900 | 2,200 | 2,450 | 2,900 |
| 5'7" | Small | 130 (126–135) | 1,700 | 1,950 | 2,200 | 2,600 |
| | Medium | 139 (132–147) | 1,800 | 2,100 | 2,350 | 2,800 |
| | Large | 149 (141–158) | 1,950 | 2,250 | 2,550 | 3,000 |
| 5'8" | Small | 135 (130–140) | 1,750 | 2,050 | 2,300 | 2,700 |
| | Medium | 143 (136–151) | 1,850 | 2,150 | 2,450 | 2,850 |
| | Large | 154 (145–163) | 2,000 | 2,300 | 2,600 | 3,100 |
| 5'9" | Small | 139 (134–144) | 1,800 | 2,100 | 2,350 | 2,800 |
| | Medium | 147 (140–155) | 1,900 | 2,200 | 2,500 | 2,950 |
| | Large | 158 (149–168) | 2,050 | 2,350 | 2,700 | 3,150 |
| 5'10" | Small | 143 (138–148) | 1,850 | 2,150 | 2,450 | 2,850 |
| | Medium | 151 (144–159) | 1,950 | 2,250 | 2,550 | 3,000 |
| | Large | 163 (153–173) | 2,100 | 2,450 | 2,750 | 3,250 |

* Table adjusted for measurement of height without shoes.
** From 1959 Metropolitan Life Insurance Company, New York City. These tables are based on 1959 rather than 1983 Metropolitan Life Insurance Company height-weight tables because the earlier tables specify lower weights, more appropriate to health-related concerns.

# Food Counter

*K*eeping track of either calories or fats is easy with the Food Counter. It lists calories and fat grams (both total fat and saturated fat) for hundreds of foods, including those found in fast-food restaurants. And if you are interested in the cholesterol and sodium counts, these are listed as well.

The Food Counter offers the following information on each food: total weight in grams, grams of total fat and saturated fatty acids, number of calories, and milligrams of cholesterol and sodium. In the "Fats and Oils" section, polyunsaturated fat is also listed in grams. When you see a dash (—) in the table, it means that information was not available on that item. When foods have only a small amount of a given nutrient, the table reads "tr," for "trace." The Food Counter was prepared using data from USDA Handbooks.

Notice that the fat content of food depends on the food itself *and* the way it is cooked. In the case of meat, it also depends on the grade and fat trim.

The foods are listed in categories:

| FOOD DESCRIPTION/PORTION | Wt. (g) | Tot. Fat (g) | Sat. Fat (g) | Cal. | Chol. (mg) | Sod. (mg) |
|---|---|---|---|---|---|---|

## MEAT, POULTRY, AND SEAFOOD

### Finfish

| FOOD DESCRIPTION/PORTION | Wt. (g) | Tot. Fat (g) | Sat. Fat (g) | Cal. | Chol. (mg) | Sod. (mg) |
|---|---|---|---|---|---|---|
| Catfish, breaded and fried (3 oz.) | 84 | 11.4 | 2.7 | 195 | 69 | 237 |
| Cod, Atlantic, cooked, dry heat (3 oz.) | 84 | 0.6 | 0.3 | 90 | 48 | 66 |
| Eel, cooked, dry heat (3 oz.) | 84 | 12.6 | 2.7 | 201 | 138 | 54 |
| Fish Sticks and portions, frozen and reheated (3 oz.) | 84 | 10.2 | 2.7 | 228 | 93 | 489 |
| Flounder, cooked, dry heat (3 oz.) | 84 | 1.2 | 0.3 | 99 | 57 | 90 |
| Grouper, cooked, dry heat (3 oz.) | 84 | 1.2 | 0.3 | 99 | 39 | 45 |
| Haddock, cooked, dry heat (3 oz.) | 84 | 0.9 | 0.3 | 96 | 63 | 75 |
| Halibut, cooked, dry heat (3 oz.) | 84 | 2.4 | 0.3 | 120 | 36 | 60 |
| Herring, pickled (3 oz.) | 84 | 15.3 | 2.1 | 222 | 12 | 741 |
| Mackerel, canned, drained solids (3 oz.) | 84 | 5.4 | 1.5 | 132 | 66 | 321 |
| Mackerel, cooked, dry heat (3 oz.) | 84 | 15.0 | 3.6 | 222 | 63 | 72 |
| Ocean Perch, cooked, dry heat (3 oz.) | 84 | 1.8 | 0.3 | 102 | 45 | 81 |
| Perch, cooked, dry heat (3 oz.) | 84 | 0.9 | 0.3 | 99 | 99 | 66 |
| Pike, Northern, cooked, dry (3 oz.) | 84 | 0.9 | tr | 96 | 42 | 42 |
| Pollack, Walleye, cooked, dry heat (3 oz.) | 84 | 0.9 | 0.3 | 96 | 81 | 99 |
| Pompano, cooked, dry heat (3 oz.) | 84 | 10.2 | 3.9 | 180 | 54 | 66 |
| Redfish (see Ocean Perch) | | | | | | |

| FOOD DESCRIPTION/PORTION | Wt. (g) | Tot. Fat (g) | Sat. Fat (g) | Cal. | Chol. (mg) | Sod. (mg) |
|---|---|---|---|---|---|---|
| Rockfish, cooked, dry heat (3 oz.) | 84 | 1.8 | 0.3 | 102 | 39 | 66 |
| Salmon, Chinook, smoked (3 oz.) | 84 | 3.6 | 0.9 | 99 | 21 | 660* |
| Salmon, Chum, canned, drained solids with bone (3 oz.) | 84 | 4.8 | 1.2 | 120 | 33 | 414** |
| Salmon, Coho, cooked, moist heat (3 oz.) | 84 | 6.3 | 1.2 | 156 | 42 | 51 |
| Salmon, Sockeye, canned, drained solids with bone (3 oz.) | 84 | 6.3 | 1.5 | 129 | 36 | 459** |
| Sardine, Atlantic, canned in oil, drained solids with bone (3 oz.) | 84 | 9.6 | tr | 177 | 120 | 429 |
| Sardine, Pacific, canned in tomato sauce, drained solids with bone (3 oz.) | 84 | 10.2 | 2.7 | 150 | 51 | 351 |
| Scrod (see Cod, page 17) | | | | | | |
| Sea Bass, cooked, dry heat (3 oz.) | 84 | 2.1 | 0.6 | 105 | 45 | 75 |
| Snapper, cooked, dry heat (3 oz.) | 84 | 1.5 | 0.3 | 108 | 39 | 48 |
| Sole (see Flounder) | | | | | | |
| Swordfish, cooked, dry heat (3 oz.) | 84 | 4.5 | 1.2 | 132 | 42 | 99 |
| Trout, Rainbow, cooked, dry heat (3 oz.) | 84 | 3.6 | 0.6 | 129 | 63 | 30 |
| Tuna, light, canned in oil, drained solids (3 oz.) | 84 | 6.9 | 1.2 | 168 | 15 | 300 |
| Tuna, light, canned in water, drained solids (3 oz.) | 84 | 0.3 | 0.3 | 111 | — | 303 |
| Tuna, white, canned in oil, drained solids (3 oz.) | 84 | 6.9 | — | 159 | 27 | 336 |

* Regular lox has approximately 567 mg sodium per ounce.
** With added salt.

| FOOD DESCRIPTION/PORTION | Wt. (g) | Tot. Fat (g) | Sat. Fat (g) | Cal. | Chol. (mg) | Sod. (mg) |
|---|---|---|---|---|---|---|
| Tuna, white, canned in water, drained solids (3 oz.) | 84 | 2.1 | 0.6 | 117 | 36 | 333 |
| Tuna Salad, prepared with light tuna in oil, pickle relish, salad dressing, onion, celery (½ cup) | 103 | 9.5 | 1.6 | 192 | 14 | 412 |

**Shellfish**

| FOOD DESCRIPTION/PORTION | Wt. (g) | Tot. Fat (g) | Sat. Fat (g) | Cal. | Chol. (mg) | Sod. (mg) |
|---|---|---|---|---|---|---|
| Clams, cooked, moist heat (3 oz.) | 84 | 1.8 | 0.3 | 126 | 57 | 96 |
| Crab, Alaskan King, cooked, moist heat (3 oz.) | 84 | 1.2 | tr | 81 | 45 | 912 |
| Crab, Alaskan King, imitation, made from surimi (3 oz.) | 84 | 1.2 | — | 87 | 18 | 714 |
| Crab, Blue, cooked, moist heat (3 oz.) | 84 | 1.5 | 0.3 | 87 | 84 | 237 |
| Crab Cakes, prepared with egg, fried in margarine (3 oz.) | 90 | 6.8 | 1.4 | 140 | 135 | 297 |
| Crayfish, cooked, moist heat (3 oz.) | 84 | 1.2 | 0.3 | 96 | 150 | 57 |
| Lobster, Northern, cooked, moist heat (3 oz.) | 84 | 0.6 | tr | 84 | 60 | 324 |
| Oysters, Eastern, breaded and fried (3 oz.) | 84 | 10.8 | 2.7 | 168 | 69 | 354 |
| Scallops, breaded and fried (6 large) | 93 | 10.2 | 2.4 | 201 | 57 | 432 |
| Shrimp, breaded and fried (12 large) | 90 | 11.1 | 1.8 | 219 | 159 | 309 |
| Shrimp, cooked (3 oz.) | 84 | 0.9 | 0.3 | 84 | 165 | 189 |
| Shrimp, imitation, made from surimi (3 oz.) | 94 | 1.2 | — | 87 | 30 | 600 |

**Chicken**

| FOOD DESCRIPTION/PORTION | Wt. (g) | Tot. Fat (g) | Sat. Fat (g) | Cal. | Chol. (mg) | Sod. (mg) |
|---|---|---|---|---|---|---|
| Light Meat, without skin, stewed (3 oz.) | 84 | 3.3 | 0.9 | 135 | 66 | 54 |

| FOOD DESCRIPTION/PORTION | Wt. (g) | Tot. Fat (g) | Sat. Fat (g) | Cal. | Chol. (mg) | Sod. (mg) |
|---|---|---|---|---|---|---|
| Light Meat, with skin, stewed (3 oz.) | 84 | 8.4 | 2.4 | 171 | 63 | 54 |
| Dark Meat, without skin, stewed (3 oz.) | 84 | 7.5 | 2.1 | 162 | 75 | 63 |
| Dark Meat, with skin, stewed (3 oz.) | 84 | 12.6 | 4.8 | 198 | 69 | 60 |
| Breast, half, meat only, stewed (3 oz.) | 95 | 2.9 | 0.8 | 144 | 73 | 59 |
| Breast, half, meat and skin, stewed (4 oz.) | 110 | 8.2 | 2.3 | 202 | 83 | 68 |
| Breast, half, meat and skin, fried with batter (5 oz.) | 140 | 18.5 | 4.9 | 364 | 119 | 385 |
| Drumstick, meat only, stewed (1½ oz.) | 46 | 2.6 | 0.7 | 78 | 40 | 37 |
| Drumstick, meat and skin, stewed (2 oz.) | 57 | 6.1 | 1.7 | 116 | 48 | 43 |
| Drumstick, meat and skin, fried with batter (2½ oz.) | 72 | 11.3 | 3.0 | 193 | 62 | 194 |
| Thigh, meat only, stewed (2 oz.) | 55 | 5.4 | 1.5 | 107 | 49 | 41 |
| Thigh, meat and skin, stewed (2½ oz.) | 68 | 10.0 | 2.8 | 158 | 57 | 49 |
| Thigh, meat and skin, fried with batter (3 oz.) | 86 | 14.2 | 3.8 | 238 | 80 | 248 |
| Wing, meat only, stewed (1 oz.) | 24 | 1.7 | 0.5 | 43 | 18 | 18 |
| Wing, meat and skin, stewed (1½ oz.) | 40 | 6.7 | 1.9 | 100 | 28 | 27 |
| Wing, meat and skin, fried with batter (1¾ oz.) | 49 | 10.7 | 2.9 | 159 | 39 | 157 |
| Boneless, canned in broth (3 oz.) | 84 | 6.6 | 1.8 | 141 | 186 | 429 |
| Frankfurter, chicken (3 oz.) | 84 | 16.5 | 4.8 | 219 | 84 | 1164 |
| Giblets—gizzard, heart, liver (1 each) (2½ oz.) | 68 | 3.6 | 1.1 | 112 | 243 | 40 |
| Giblets—gizzard, heart, liver (3 oz.) | 84 | 4.5 | 1.5 | 141 | 303 | 51 |

| FOOD DESCRIPTION/PORTION | Wt. (g) | Tot. Fat (g) | Sat. Fat (g) | Cal. | Chol. (mg) | Sod. (mg) |
|---|---|---|---|---|---|---|
| Liver Pâté, canned | | | | | | |
| (6 Tbsp.) | 84 | 11.1 | — | 171 | — | — |
| Chicken Roll, light (3 oz.) | 84 | 6.3 | 1.8 | 135 | 42 | 498 |
| Spread, canned (3 oz.) | 84 | 9.9 | — | 165 | — | — |
| | | | | | | |
| **Turkey** | | | | | | |
| Light Meat, meat only, | | | | | | |
| roasted (3 oz.) | 84 | 0.9 | 0.3 | 120 | 72 | 48 |
| Light Meat, meat and skin, | | | | | | |
| roasted (3 oz.) | 84 | 7.2 | 2.1 | 138 | 66 | 54 |
| Dark Meat, meat only, | | | | | | |
| roasted (3 oz.) | 84 | 3.6 | 1.2 | 138 | 96 | 66 |
| Dark Meat, meat and skin, | | | | | | |
| roasted (3 oz.) | 84 | 9.9 | 3.0 | 189 | 75 | 66 |
| Turkey Ham, cured, thigh | | | | | | |
| meat (3 oz.) | 84 | 4.2 | 1.5 | 111 | — | 849 |
| Turkey Pastrami (3 oz.) | 84 | 5.4 | 1.5 | 120 | — | 891 |
| Turkey Roll, light and dark | | | | | | |
| meat (3 oz.) | 84 | 6.0 | 1.8 | 126 | 48 | 498 |
| Turkey, frozen with gravy, | | | | | | |
| 1 package (15 oz.) | 426 | 11.1 | 3.6 | 285 | — | 2358 |
| Turkey, frozen with gravy | | | | | | |
| (3 oz.) | 84 | 2.4 | 0.6 | 57 | — | 471 |
| Giblets—gizzard, heart, | | | | | | |
| liver (1 each) (5½ oz.) | 158 | 8.0 | 2.4 | 264 | 660 | 92 |
| Giblets—gizzard, heart, | | | | | | |
| liver (3 oz.) | 84 | 4.2 | 1.2 | 141 | 357 | 51 |
| Young Toms, meat only, | | | | | | |
| roasted (3 oz.) | 84 | 3.9 | 1.3 | 141 | 65 | 62 |
| Young Toms, light meat | | | | | | |
| without skin, roasted | | | | | | |
| (3 oz.) | 84 | 2.4 | 0.8 | 129 | 58 | 57 |
| | | | | | | |
| **Beef** | | | | | | |
| Arm Pot Roast, choice, lean | | | | | | |
| only, trimmed to 0″ fat, | | | | | | |
| braised (3 oz.) | 85 | 7.4 | 2.7 | 187 | 86 | 56 |

| FOOD DESCRIPTION/PORTION | Wt. (g) | Tot. Fat (g) | Sat. Fat (g) | Cal. | Chol. (mg) | Sod. (mg) |
|---|---|---|---|---|---|---|
| Arm Pot Roast, choice, lean only, trimmed to ¼″ fat, braised (3 oz.) | 85 | 7.9 | 2.9 | 191 | 86 | 56 |
| Arm Pot Roast, select, lean only, trimmed to 0″ fat, braised (3 oz.) | 85 | 5.4 | 1.9 | 168 | 86 | 56 |
| Arm Pot Roast, select, lean only, trimmed to ¼″ fat, braised (3 oz.) | 85 | 6.1 | 2.2 | 175 | 86 | 56 |
| Blade Roast, choice, lean and fat, trimmed to ¼″ fat, braised (3 oz.) | 85 | 23.7 | 9.3 | 309 | 88 | 54 |
| Blade Roast, choice, lean only, trimmed to 0″ fat, braised (3 oz.) | 85 | 12.5 | 4.9 | 225 | 90 | 60 |
| Blade Roast, choice, lean only, trimmed to ¼″ fat, braised (3 oz.) | 85 | 12.2 | 4.8 | 223 | 90 | 60 |
| Bottom Round, choice, lean only, trimmed to 0″ fat, braised (3 oz.) | 85 | 7.4 | 2.5 | 181 | 82 | 43 |
| Bottom Round, choice, lean only, trimmed to ¼″ fat, braised (3 oz.) | 85 | 8.0 | 2.7 | 187 | 82 | 43 |
| Bottom Round, choice, lean only, trimmed to 0″ fat, roasted (3 oz.) | 85 | 6.6 | 2.2 | 164 | 66 | 56 |
| Bottom Round, choice, lean only, trimmed to ¼″ fat, roasted (3 oz.) | 85 | 7.1 | 2.4 | 168 | 66 | 56 |
| Bottom Round, select, lean only, trimmed to 0″ fat, braised (3 oz.) | 85 | 5.4 | 1.8 | 163 | 82 | 43 |
| Bottom Round, select, lean only, trimmed to ¼″ fat, braised (3 oz.) | 85 | 5.8 | 2.0 | 167 | 82 | 43 |

| FOOD DESCRIPTION/PORTION | Wt. (g) | Tot. Fat (g) | Sat. Fat (g) | Cal. | Chol. (mg) | Sod. (mg) |
|---|---|---|---|---|---|---|
| Bottom Round, select, lean only, trimmed to 0″ fat, roasted (3 oz.) | 85 | 4.6 | 1.5 | 146 | 66 | 56 |
| Bottom Round, select, lean only, trimmed to ¼″ fat, roasted (3 oz.) | 85 | 5.3 | 1.8 | 152 | 66 | 56 |
| Eye of Round, choice, lean only, trimmed to 0″ fat, roasted (3 oz.) | 85 | 4.8 | 1.8 | 149 | 59 | 53 |
| Eye of Round, select, lean only, trimmed to 0″ fat, roasted (3 oz.) | 85 | 3.0 | 1.1 | 132 | 59 | 53 |
| Eye of Round, select, lean only, trimmed to ¼″ fat, roasted (3 oz.) | 85 | 3.4 | 1.2 | 136 | 59 | 53 |
| Flank, choice, lean only, trimmed to 0″ fat, broiled (3 oz.) | 85 | 8.7 | 3 6 | 177 | 57 | 70 |
| Ground, extra lean, broiled, medium (3 oz.) | 85 | 13.9 | 5.5 | 217 | 71 | 59 |
| Ground, lean, broiled, medium (3 oz.) | 85 | 15.7 | 6.2 | 231 | 74 | 65 |
| Ground, regular, broiled, medium (3 oz.) | 85 | 17.7 | 6.9 | 246 | 76 | 70 |
| Heart, simmered (3 oz.) | 85 | 4.8 | 1.5 | 147 | 165 | 54 |
| Kidney, simmered (3 oz.) | 85 | 3.0 | 0.9 | 123 | 330 | 114 |
| Liver, braised (3 oz.) | 85 | 4.2 | 1.5 | 138 | 330 | 90 |
| Rib, large end (ribs 6–9), choice, lean only, trimmed to 0″ fat, roasted (3 oz.) | 85 | 12.9 | 5.1 | 216 | 69 | 62 |
| Rib, large end (ribs 6–9), choice, lean and fat, trimmed to 0″ fat, roasted (3 oz.) | 85 | 26.0 | 10.5 | 317 | 72 | 54 |

| FOOD DESCRIPTION/PORTION | Wt. (g) | Tot. Fat (g) | Sat. Fat (g) | Cal. | Chol. (mg) | Sod. (mg) |
|---|---|---|---|---|---|---|
| Rib, large end (ribs 6–9), choice, lean and fat, trimmed to ¼″ fat, roasted (3 oz.) | 85 | 27.3 | 11.1 | 327 | 73 | 54 |
| Rib, small end (ribs 10–12), choice, lean only, trimmed to 0″ fat, broiled (3 oz.) | 85 | 9.9 | 3.9 | 192 | 68 | 59 |
| Rib, small end (ribs 10–12), choice, lean only, trimmed to ¼″ fat, broiled (3 oz.) | 85 | 10.7 | 4.3 | 198 | 68 | 59 |
| Rib, small end (ribs 10–12), choice, lean and fat, trimmed to ¼″ fat, broiled (3 oz.) | 85 | 23.4 | 9.6 | 297 | 71 | 52 |
| Rib, small end, select, lean only, trimmed to 0″ fat, broiled (3 oz.) | 85 | 7.4 | 3.0 | 168 | 68 | 59 |
| Rib, small end, select, lean only, trimmed to ¼″ fat, broiled (3 oz.) | 85 | 8.2 | 3.3 | 176 | 68 | 59 |
| Rib, whole, select, lean only, trimmed to ¼″ fat, broiled (3 oz.) | 85 | 8.9 | 3.6 | 175 | 66 | 60 |
| T-Bone Steak, choice, lean only, trimmed to ¼″ fat, broiled (3 oz.) | 85 | 8.8 | 3.5 | 182 | 68 | 56 |
| Tenderloin, choice, lean only, trimmed to 0″ fat, broiled (3 oz.) | 85 | 8.6 | 3.2 | 180 | 71 | 54 |
| Tenderloin, choice, lean only, trimmed to ¼″ fat, broiled (3 oz.) | 85 | 9.5 | 3.6 | 188 | 71 | 54 |

| FOOD DESCRIPTION/PORTION | Wt. (g) | Tot. Fat (g) | Sat. Fat (g) | Cal. | Chol. (mg) | Sod. (mg) |
|---|---|---|---|---|---|---|
| Tenderloin, select, lean only, trimmed to 0″ fat, broiled (3 oz.) | 85 | 7.5 | 2.8 | 170 | 71 | 54 |
| Tip Round, choice, lean only, trimmed to 0″ fat, roasted (3 oz.) | 85 | 5.4 | 1.9 | 153 | 69 | 55 |
| Tip Round, choice, lean only, trimmed to ¼″ fat, roasted (3 oz.) | 85 | 6.2 | 2.2 | 160 | 69 | 55 |
| Tip Round, select, lean and fat, trimmed to 0″ fat, roasted (3 oz.) | 85 | 6.2 | 2.3 | 158 | 69 | 55 |
| Tip Round, select, lean only, trimmed to ¼″ fat, roasted (3 oz.) | 85 | 5.4 | 1.9 | 153 | 69 | 55 |
| Tongue, simmered (3 oz.) | 85 | 17.7 | 7.5 | 240 | 90 | 51 |
| Top Loin, choice, lean only, trimmed to 0″ fat, broiled (3 oz.) | 85 | 8.2 | 3.1 | 177 | 65 | 58 |
| Top Loin, choice, lean only, trimmed to ¼″ fat, broiled (3 oz.) | 85 | 8.6 | 3.3 | 182 | 65 | 58 |
| Top Loin, select, lean only, trimmed to 0″ fat, broiled (3 oz.) | 85 | 5.9 | 2.2 | 157 | 65 | 58 |
| Top Loin, select, lean only, trimmed to ¼″ fat, broiled (3 oz.) | 85 | 6.6 | 2.5 | 164 | 65 | 58 |
| Top Round, choice, lean only, trimmed to 0″ fat, braised (3 oz.) | 85 | 4.9 | 1.7 | 176 | 76 | 38 |
| Top Round, choice, lean only, trimmed to ¼″ fat, braised (3 oz.) | 85 | 5.5 | 1.9 | 181 | 76 | 38 |
| Top Round, choice, lean only, trimmed to ¼″ fat, broiled (3 oz.) | 85 | 5.0 | 1.7 | 160 | 71 | 52 |

| FOOD DESCRIPTION/PORTION | Wt. (g) | Tot. Fat (g) | Sat. Fat (g) | Cal. | Chol. (mg) | Sod. (mg) |
|---|---|---|---|---|---|---|
| Top Round, choice, lean only, trimmed to ¼″ fat, pan-fried (3 oz.) | 85 | 7.3 | 2.1 | 193 | 82 | 60 |
| Top Round, select, lean only, trimmed to 0″ fat, braised (3 oz.) | 85 | 3.4 | 1.2 | 162 | 76 | 38 |
| Top Round, select, lean only, trimmed to ¼″ fat, braised (3 oz.) | 85 | 3.9 | 1.3 | 166 | 76 | 38 |
| Top Round, select, lean only, trimmed to ¼″ fat, broiled (3 oz.) | 85 | 3.1 | 1.1 | 143 | 71 | 52 |
| Top Sirloin, choice, lean only, trimmed to 0″ fat, broiled (3 oz.) | 85 | 6.6 | 2.6 | 170 | 76 | 56 |
| Top Sirloin, choice, lean only, trimmed to ¼″ fat, broiled (3 oz.) | 85 | 6.8 | 2.7 | 172 | 76 | 56 |
| Top Sirloin, select, lean only, trimmed to 0″ fat, broiled (3 oz.) | 85 | 4.8 | 1.9 | 153 | 76 | 56 |
| Top Sirloin, select, lean only, trimmed to ¼″ fat, broiled (3 oz.) | 85 | 5.3 | 2.1 | 158 | 76 | 56 |
| Tripe (3 oz.) | 85 | 3.3 | 1.8 | 84 | 81 | 39 |
| **Veal** | | | | | | |
| Arm Steak, lean only, braised (3 oz.) | 84 | 4.5 | 1.2 | 171 | 132 | 75 |
| Average, all grades, lean only, cooked (3 oz.) | 84 | 5.7 | 1.5 | 165 | 99 | 75 |
| Blade Steak, lean only, braised (3 oz.) | 84 | 5.4 | 1.5 | 168 | 135 | 87 |
| Loin Chop, lean only, braised (3 oz.) | 84 | 6.0 | 2.1 | 150 | 90 | 81 |
| Rib Roast, lean only, cooked (3 oz.) | 84 | 6.3 | 1.8 | 150 | 96 | 81 |

| FOOD DESCRIPTION/PORTION | Wt. (g) | Tot. Fat (g) | Sat. Fat (g) | Cal. | Chol. (mg) | Sod. (mg) |
|---|---|---|---|---|---|---|
| **Lamb** | | | | | | |
| Average, all grades, lean only, cooked (3 oz.) | 84 | 8.1 | 3.0 | 174 | 78 | 63 |
| Foreshank, lean only, braised (3 oz.) | 84 | 5.1 | 1.8 | 159 | 90 | 63 |
| Leg, shank portion, lean only, roasted (3 oz.) | 84 | 5.7 | 2.1 | 153 | 75 | 57 |
| Loin Chops, lean only, broiled (3 oz.) | 84 | 8.4 | 1.8 | 183 | 81 | 72 |
| Rack, rib, lean only, roasted (3 oz.) | 84 | 11.4 | 3.9 | 198 | 75 | 69 |
| **Pork** | | | | | | |
| Bacon, pan-fried, 4½ slices (1 oz.) | 28 | 14.0 | 5.0 | 163 | 24 | 452 |
| Canadian Bacon, grilled (3 oz.) | 84 | 7.2 | 2.4 | 156 | 48 | 1314 |
| Chitterlings, simmered (3 oz.) | 84 | 24.6 | 8.7 | 258 | 123 | 33 |
| Fresh Pork, center loin, lean only, broiled (3 oz.) | 84 | 9.0 | 3.0 | 195 | 84 | 66 |
| Fresh Pork, arm, picnic, shoulder, lean only, roasted (3 oz.) | 84 | 10.8 | 3.6 | 195 | 81 | 69 |
| Fresh Pork, shoulder, blade, Boston, lean only, roasted (3 oz.) | 84 | 14.4 | 4.8 | 219 | 84 | 63 |
| Fresh Pork, sirloin, lean only, broiled (3 oz.) | 84 | 11.7 | 3.9 | 207 | 84 | 51 |
| Fresh Pork, tenderloin, lean only, roasted (3 oz.) | 84 | 4.2 | 1.5 | 141 | 78 | 57 |
| Fresh Pork, whole leg, lean only, roasted (3 oz.) | 84 | 9.3 | 3.3 | 186 | 81 | 54 |
| Ham, boneless, canned, extra lean, roasted (3 oz.) | 84 | 4.2 | 1.5 | 117 | 24 | 966 |

| FOOD DESCRIPTION/PORTION | Wt. (g) | Tot. Fat (g) | Sat. Fat (g) | Cal. | Chol. (mg) | Sod. (mg) |
|---|---|---|---|---|---|---|
| Ham, boneless, canned, regular, roasted (3 oz.) | 84 | 12.9 | 4.2 | 192 | 51 | 801 |
| Ham, boneless, extra lean, roasted (3 oz.) | 84 | 4.8 | 1.5 | 123 | 45 | 1023 |
| Liver, braised (3 oz.) | 84 | 3.9 | 1.2 | 141 | 303 | 42 |
| Spareribs, lean and fat, braised (3 oz.) | 84 | 25.8 | 9.9 | 339 | 102 | 78 |
| **Game** | | | | | | |
| Deer (Venison), roasted (3 oz.) | 85 | 2.7 | 1.1 | 134 | 95 | 46 |
| Goose, domesticated, meat only, roasted (3 oz.) | 84 | 10.8 | 3.9 | 201 | 78 | 60 |
| Goose, domesticated, meat and skin, roasted (3 oz.) | 84 | 18.6 | 6.0 | 258 | 78 | 60 |
| Rabbit, domesticated, stewed (3 oz.) | 85 | 7.2 | 2.1 | 175 | 73 | 31 |
| **Luncheon Meat and Sausage** | | | | | | |
| Bologna, beef and pork (3 oz.) | 84 | 24.0 | 9.0 | 267 | 48 | 867 |
| Braunschweiger, pork (3 oz.) | 84 | 27.3 | 9.3 | 306 | 132 | 972 |
| Chicken Spread, canned (6 Tbsp.) | 78 | 9.9 | — | 165 | — | — |
| Frankfurter, beef and pork (3 oz.) | 84 | 24.9 | 9.3 | 273 | 42 | 954 |
| Frankfurter, chicken (3 oz.) | 84 | 16.5 | 4.8 | 219 | 84 | 1164 |
| Pepperoni, pork, beef (3 oz.) | 84 | 37.5 | 13.8 | 423 | — | 1734 |
| Salad Spread, ham, cured (6 Tbsp.) | 90 | 14.1 | 4.5 | 192 | 36 | 822 |
| Salami, dry, pork, beef (3 oz.) | 84 | 29.4 | 10.5 | 357 | 66 | 1581 |
| Sausage, Italian, pork, cooked (3 oz.) | 84 | 21.9 | 7.8 | 276 | 66 | 783 |

| FOOD DESCRIPTION/PORTION | Wt. (g) | Tot. Fat (g) | Sat. Fat (g) | Cal. | Chol. (mg) | Sod. (mg) |
|---|---|---|---|---|---|---|
| Sausage, knockwurst, pork, beef (3 oz.) | 84 | 23.7 | 8.7 | 261 | 48 | 858 |
| Sausage, liverwurst, pork (3 oz.) | 84 | 24.3 | 9.0 | 279 | 135 | 732 |
| Sausage, Polish, pork (3 oz.) | 84 | 24.3 | 8.7 | 276 | 60 | 744 |
| Sausage, pork, fresh, cooked (3 oz.) | 84 | 26.4 | 9.3 | 315 | 72 | 1098 |
| Sausage, Vienna, beef and pork, canned (4½ links) | 84 | 21.3 | 7.8 | 237 | 45 | 810 |

**Mixed Dishes with Meat, Poultry, and Seafood**

| FOOD DESCRIPTION/PORTION | Wt. (g) | Tot. Fat (g) | Sat. Fat (g) | Cal. | Chol. (mg) | Sod. (mg) |
|---|---|---|---|---|---|---|
| Chicken à la King (1 cup) | 245 | 34.3 | 12.9 | 468 | 220 | 760 |
| Chicken and Noodle Casserole (1 cup) | 240 | 18.5 | 5.9 | 367 | — | 600 |
| Chili con Carne, with beans, canned (1 cup) | 255 | 14.0 | 6.0 | 286 | — | 1330 |
| Chop Suey, beef and pork, without noodles (1 cup) | 250 | 17.0 | 8.5 | 300 | — | 1053 |
| Chow Mein, chicken, without noodles (1 cup) | 250 | 10.0 | 2.4 | 255 | — | 718 |
| Macaroni and Cheese, canned (1 cup) | 240 | 9.6 | 4.2 | 228 | — | 730 |
| Macaroni and Cheese, homemade (1 cup) | 200 | 22.2 | 11.9 | 430 | — | 1086 |
| Pâté, chicken liver (½ cup) | 104 | 13.6 | — | 208 | — | 0 |
| Pizza, cheese (⅛ of 12″ diameter) | 49 | 2.5 | 1.2 | 109 | 7 | 261 |
| Pizza, cheese, pepperoni (⅛ of 12″ diameter) | 53 | 5.2 | 1.7 | 135 | 11 | 199 |
| Pot Pie, beef (⅓ of 9″ diameter) | 210 | 30.5 | 7.9 | 517 | 42 | 596 |
| Pot Pie, chicken (⅓ of 9″ diameter) | 232 | 31.3 | 10.3 | 545 | 56 | 594 |
| Spaghetti, with meatballs and tomato sauce, canned (1 cup) | 250 | 10.8 | 2.2 | 258 | — | 1220 |

| FOOD DESCRIPTION/PORTION | Wt. (g) | Tot. Fat (g) | Sat. Fat (g) | Cal. | Chol. (mg) | Sod. (mg) |
|---|---|---|---|---|---|---|
| Stew, beef and vegetables (1 cup) | 245 | 10.5 | 4.4 | 218 | 72 | 292 |

## FAST FOOD

| FOOD DESCRIPTION/PORTION | Wt. (g) | Tot. Fat (g) | Sat. Fat (g) | Cal. | Chol. (mg) | Sod. (mg) |
|---|---|---|---|---|---|---|
| Bacon Cheeseburger, single patty with condiments (1) | 195 | 36.8 | 16.3 | 609 | 112 | 1044 |
| Burrito, with beans (2) | 217 | 13.5 | 6.9 | 448 | 5 | 986 |
| Burrito, with beans, cheese and beef (2) | 203 | 13.3 | 7.2 | 331 | 125 | 990 |
| Cheeseburger, large, single meat patty, plain (1) | 185 | 33.0 | 14.8 | 608 | 96 | 1589 |
| Cheeseburger, large, single meat patty with condiments and vegetables (1) | 219 | 32.9 | 15.0 | 564 | 88 | 1107 |
| Cheeseburger, regular, single meat patty with condiments (1) | 113 | 14.1 | 6.3 | 295 | 37 | 616 |
| Chicken, breaded and fried, light meat (breast or wing) (2 pieces) | 163 | 29.5 | 7.8 | 494 | 149 | 975 |
| Chicken Fillet Sandwich, plain (1) | 182 | 29.5 | 8.5 | 515 | 60 | 957 |
| Chimichanga, with beef (1) | 174 | 19.7 | 8.5 | 425 | 9 | 910 |
| Cookies, animal crackers (1 box) | 67 | 9.0 | 3.5 | 299 | 11 | 274 |
| Eggs, scrambled (2) | 94 | 15.2 | 5.8 | 200 | 400 | 211 |
| Enchilada, with cheese and beef (1) | 192 | 17.6 | 9.1 | 324 | 40 | 1320 |
| English Muffin Sandwich with egg, cheese, Canadian bacon (1) | 146 | 19.8 | 9.1 | 383 | 234 | 785 |
| Fish Sandwich, with tartar sauce (1) | 158 | 22.8 | 5.2 | 431 | 55 | 615 |

| FOOD DESCRIPTION/PORTION | Wt. (g) | Tot. Fat (g) | Sat. Fat (g) | Cal. | Chol. (mg) | Sod. (mg) |
|---|---|---|---|---|---|---|
| Fish Sandwich, with tartar sauce and cheese (1) | 183 | 28.6 | 8.1 | 524 | 68 | 939 |
| Fried Pie, apple, cherry or lemon (1) | 85 | 14.4 | 6.5 | 266 | 13 | 325 |
| Ham and Cheese Sandwich (1) | 146 | 15.5 | 6.4 | 353 | 58 | 772 |
| Hamburger, double meat, with condiments (1) | 215 | 32.5 | 12.0 | 576 | 102 | 742 |
| Hamburger, large, single meat patty with condiments and vegetables (1) | 218 | 27.4 | 10.4 | 511 | 86 | 825 |
| Hamburger, large, triple meat patty, plain, with condiments (1) | 259 | 41.5 | 15.9 | 693 | 142 | 713 |
| Hamburger, regular, single meat patty, plain (1) | 90 | 11.8 | 4.1 | 275 | 36 | 387 |
| Hamburger, regular, single meat patty with condiments and vegetables (1) | 110 | 13.5 | 4.1 | 279 | 26 | 504 |
| Hot Dog (1) | 98 | 14.5 | 5.1 | 242 | 44 | 671 |
| Hot Fudge Sundae (1) | 158 | 8.6 | 5.0 | 284 | 21 | 182 |
| Hush Puppies (5 pieces) | 78 | 11.6 | 2.7 | 256 | 135 | 965 |
| Onion Rings (8–9 rings) | 83 | 15.5 | 7.0 | 275 | 14 | 430 |
| Pancake, with butter and syrup (3) | 232 | 14.0 | 5.9 | 519 | 57 | 1103 |
| Potato, french-fried in beef tallow and vegetable oil (4 oz.) | 115 | 18.5 | 7.6 | 358 | 16 | 187 |
| Potato, french-fried in vegetable oil (1 regular order) | 76 | 12.2 | 3.8 | 235 | 0 | 124 |
| Potato Chips (10) | 20 | 7.1 | 1.8 | 105 | — | 94 |
| Roast Beef, on bun (1) | 139 | 13.8 | 3.6 | 346 | 52 | 792 |

| FOOD DESCRIPTION/PORTION | Wt. (g) | Tot. Fat (g) | Sat. Fat (g) | Cal. | Chol. (mg) | Sod. (mg) |
|---|---|---|---|---|---|---|
| Shake, chocolate | | | | | | |
| (10 fluid oz.) | 283 | 10.5 | 6.5 | 360 | 37 | 273 |
| Taco, small (1) | 171 | 20.6 | 11.4 | 370 | 57 | 802 |
| Tuna Salad Sub (1) | 256 | 28.0 | 5.3 | 584 | 47 | 1294 |

## EGGS

| FOOD DESCRIPTION/PORTION | Wt. (g) | Tot. Fat (g) | Sat. Fat (g) | Cal. | Chol. (mg) | Sod. (mg) |
|---|---|---|---|---|---|---|
| Egg, whole, raw (1) | 50 | 5.0 | 1.6 | 75 | 213 | 63 |
| Egg White, raw (1) | 33 | tr | 0 | 16 | 0 | 50 |
| Egg Yolk, raw (1) | 17 | 5.0 | 1.6 | 63 | 213 | 8 |
| Egg, fried in butter (1) | 46 | 6.4 | 2.4 | 83 | 219 | 144 |
| Egg, scrambled with butter | | | | | | |
| and milk (1 egg) | 64 | 7.1 | 2.8 | 95 | 225 | 155 |
| Egg Substitute, frozen | | | | | | |
| (¼ cup) | 60 | 6.7 | 1.2 | 96 | 1 | 120 |
| Egg Substitute,* liquid (¼ cup) | 60 | 2.0 | 0.4 | 50 | 1 | 106 |
| Omelet, with butter and | | | | | | |
| milk (1 egg) | 64 | 7.1 | 2.8 | 95 | 225 | 155 |

## MILK PRODUCTS

| FOOD DESCRIPTION/PORTION | Wt. (g) | Tot. Fat (g) | Sat. Fat (g) | Cal. | Chol. (mg) | Sod. (mg) |
|---|---|---|---|---|---|---|
| Buttermilk, cultured (1 cup) | 245 | 2.2 | 1.3 | 99 | 9 | 257 |
| Condensed, sweetened, | | | | | | |
| canned (1 cup) | 306 | 26.6 | 16.8 | 982 | 104 | 389 |
| Evaporated, skim, canned | | | | | | |
| (½ cup) | 128 | 0.3 | 0.2 | 99 | 5 | 147 |
| Evaporated, whole, canned | | | | | | |
| (½ cup) | 126 | 9.5 | 5.8 | 169 | 37 | 133 |
| Hot Cocoa, with whole milk | | | | | | |
| (1 cup) | 250 | 9.1 | 5.6 | 218 | 33 | 123 |
| Malted Milk Beverage | | | | | | |
| (1 cup whole milk + 4 | | | | | | |
| to 5 heaping tsp. | | | | | | |
| malted milk powder) | 265 | 8.9 | 5.5 | 225 | 33 | 244 |

* Check labels—several brands are fat-free.

| FOOD DESCRIPTION/PORTION | Wt. (g) | Tot. Fat (g) | Sat. Fat (g) | Cal. | Chol. (mg) | Sod. (mg) |
|---|---|---|---|---|---|---|
| Milk, skim or nonfat (1 cup) | 245 | 0.4 | 0.3 | 86 | 4 | 126 |
| Milk, 1% fat (1 cup) | 244 | 2.6 | 1.6 | 102 | 10 | 123 |
| Milk, 2% fat (1 cup) | 244 | 4.7 | 2.9 | 121 | 18 | 122 |
| Milk, whole (1 cup) | 244 | 8.2 | 5.1 | 150 | 33 | 120 |
| Milk, whole, chocolate (1 cup) | 250 | 8.5 | 5.3 | 208 | 30 | 149 |
| Milkshake, vanilla, thick (11 oz.) | 313 | 9.5 | 5.9 | 350 | 37 | 299 |

**Yogurt**

| FOOD DESCRIPTION/PORTION | Wt. (g) | Tot. Fat (g) | Sat. Fat (g) | Cal. | Chol. (mg) | Sod. (mg) |
|---|---|---|---|---|---|---|
| Low-fat, plain (1 cup) | 227 | 3.5 | 2.3 | 144 | 14 | 159 |
| Nonfat or Skim, plain (1 cup) | 227 | 0.4 | 0.3 | 127 | 4 | 174 |
| Whole, plain (1 cup) | 227 | 7.4 | 4.8 | 139 | 29 | 105 |

**Frozen Desserts**

| FOOD DESCRIPTION/PORTION | Wt. (g) | Tot. Fat (g) | Sat. Fat (g) | Cal. | Chol. (mg) | Sod. (mg) |
|---|---|---|---|---|---|---|
| Frozen Yogurt (3/4 cup) | 170 | 3.5 | 2.3 | 185 | 14 | 90 |
| Ice Cream, rich, 16% fat (3/4 cup) | 111 | 17.7 | 11.1 | 263 | 66 | 81 |
| Ice Cream, regular, 10% fat (3/4 cup) | 101 | 10.7 | 6.8 | 203 | 45 | 87 |
| Ice Milk, regular (3/4 cup) | 99 | 4.2 | 2.7 | 138 | 14 | 80 |
| Ice Milk, soft serve (3/4 cup) | 132 | 3.5 | 2.1 | 168 | 11 | 123 |
| Sherbet, orange (3/4 cup) | 146 | 2.9 | 1.8 | 203 | 11 | 66 |

**Cream, Nondairy Creamers and Toppers**

| FOOD DESCRIPTION/PORTION | Wt. (g) | Tot. Fat (g) | Sat. Fat (g) | Cal. | Chol. (mg) | Sod. (mg) |
|---|---|---|---|---|---|---|
| Creamer, nondairy, liquid (2 Tbsp.) | 30 | 3.0 | 0.6 | 40 | 0 | 24 |
| Creamer, nondairy, powder (2 tsp.) | 4 | 1.4 | 1.4 | 22 | 0 | 8 |
| Dessert Topping, nondairy, frozen (2 Tbsp.) | 8 | 2.0 | 1.8 | 26 | 0 | 2 |
| Half-and-Half Cream (2 Tbsp.) | 30 | 3.4 | 2.2 | 40 | 12 | 12 |
| Sour Cream, real (2 Tbsp.) | 24 | 5.0 | 3.2 | 52 | 10 | 12 |
| Whipped Cream, pressurized (2 Tbsp.) | 6 | 1.4 | 0.8 | 16 | 4 | 8 |

| FOOD DESCRIPTION/PORTION | Wt. (g) | Tot. Fat (g) | Sat. Fat (g) | Cal. | Chol. (mg) | Sod. (mg) |
|---|---|---|---|---|---|---|
| Whipping Cream, heavy, fluid (2 Tbsp.) | 30 | 11.2 | 7.0 | 104 | 42 | 12 |
| **Cheese*** | | | | | | |
| American (1 oz.) | 28 | 8.9 | 5.6 | 106 | 27 | 406 |
| Blue, Brie, Cheddar, Colby, Edam, Gouda, Gruyère, Monterey, Parmesan, Roquefort, Swiss (1 oz.) | 28 | 9.4 | 6.0 | 114 | 30 | 176 |
| Cheese Spread, process, American (1 oz.) | 28 | 6.0 | 3.8 | 82 | 16 | 381 |
| Cottage Cheese, creamed (½ cup) | 105 | 4.7 | 3.0 | 109 | 16 | 425 |
| Cottage Cheese, dry curd (½ cup) | 73 | 0.3 | 0.2 | 62 | 5 | 10 |
| Cottage Cheese, low-fat, 1% (½ cup) | 113 | 1.2 | 0.7 | 82 | 5 | 459 |
| Cottage Cheese, low-fat, 2% (½ cup) | 113 | 2.2 | 1.4 | 101 | 9 | 459 |
| Cream Cheese, Neufchâtel (1 oz.) | 28 | 6.6 | 4.2 | 74 | 22 | 113 |
| Cream Cheese, regular (1 oz.) | 28 | 9.9 | 6.2 | 99 | 31 | 84 |
| Mozzarella, part skim (1 oz.) | 28 | 4.5 | 2.9 | 72 | 16 | 132 |
| Ricotta, part skim (1 oz.) | 28 | 2.2 | 1.4 | 39 | 9 | 35 |
| Ricotta, whole milk (1 oz.) | 28 | 3.7 | 2.4 | 49 | 14 | 24 |

* Many low-fat varieties are in grocery stores; check labels.

| FOOD DESCRIPTION/PORTION | Wt. (g) | Tot. Fat (g) | Sat. Fat (g) | Poly. Fat (g) | Cal. | Chol. (mg) | Sod. (mg) |
|---|---|---|---|---|---|---|---|

## FATS AND OILS

### Oils

| FOOD DESCRIPTION/PORTION | Wt. (g) | Tot. Fat (g) | Sat. Fat (g) | Poly. Fat (g) | Cal. | Chol. (mg) | Sod. (mg) |
|---|---|---|---|---|---|---|---|
| Canola (3 tsp.) | 15 | 13.5 | 0.9 | 4.5 | 120 | 0 | 0 |
| Corn (3 tsp.) | 15 | 13.5 | 1.8 | 8.1 | 120 | 0 | 0 |
| Olive (3 tsp.) | 15 | 13.5 | 1.8 | 1.2 | 120 | 0 | 0 |
| Peanut (3 tsp.) | 15 | 13.5 | 2.4 | 4.2 | 120 | 0 | 0 |
| Safflower (3 tsp.) | 15 | 13.5 | 1.2 | 10.2 | 120 | 0 | 0 |
| Sesame (3 tsp.) | 15 | 13.5 | 1.8 | 5.7 | 120 | 0 | 0 |
| Soybean (3 tsp.) | 15 | 13.5 | 2.1 | 7.8 | 120 | 0 | 0 |
| Soybean, hydrogenated (3 tsp.) | 15 | 13.5 | 2.1 | 5.1 | 120 | 0 | 0 |
| Soybean/Cottonseed (3 tsp.) | 15 | 13.5 | 2.4 | 6.6 | 120 | 0 | 0 |
| Sunflower (3 tsp.) | 15 | 13.5 | 1.5 | 9.0 | 120 | 0 | 0 |

### Margarines

| FOOD DESCRIPTION/PORTION | Wt. (g) | Tot. Fat (g) | Sat. Fat (g) | Poly. Fat (g) | Cal. | Chol. (mg) | Sod. (mg) |
|---|---|---|---|---|---|---|---|
| Corn Oil, stick (3 tsp.) | 15 | 11.4 | 1.8 | 2.4 | 102 | 0 | 132 |
| Corn Oil, tub (3 tsp.) | 15 | 11.4 | 2.1 | 4.5 | 102 | 0 | 153 |
| Diet (6 tsp.) | 30 | 11.4 | 1.8 | 4.8 | 99 | 0 | 276 |
| Safflower Oil, tub (3 tsp.) | 15 | 11.4 | 1.2 | 6.3 | 102 | 0 | 153 |
| Soybean, hydrogenated, tub (3 tsp.) | 15 | 11.4 | 1.8 | 3.9 | 102 | 0 | 153 |
| Soybean, hydrogenated, whipped, tub (3 tsp.) | 15 | 8.7 | 1.8 | 0.9 | 78 | 0 | 144 |

### Nuts (approximately 4½ Tbsp.)

| FOOD DESCRIPTION/PORTION | Wt. (g) | Tot. Fat (g) | Sat. Fat (g) | Poly. Fat (g) | Cal. | Chol. (mg) | Sod. (mg) |
|---|---|---|---|---|---|---|---|
| Almonds, dried | 42 | 22.2 | 2.1 | 4.7 | 251 | 0 | 5 |
| Brazil Nuts, dried | 42 | 28.2 | 6.9 | 10.4 | 279 | 0 | 0 |
| Cashews, dry-roasted | 42 | 19.8 | 3.9 | 3.3 | 245 | 0 | 6 |
| Chestnuts, roasted | 42 | 0.5 | 0.2 | 0.2 | 102 | 0 | 2 |
| Coconut, flaked, sweetened | 42 | 13.5 | 12.0 | 0.2 | 189 | 0 | 114 |
| Filberts/Hazelnuts, dried | 42 | 26.7 | 2.0 | 2.6 | 269 | 0 | 2 |
| Macadamia, oil-roasted | 42 | 32.6 | 5.0 | 0.6 | 306 | 0 | 3 |
| Mixed, dry-roasted | 42 | 21.9 | 3.0 | 4.7 | 254 | 0 | 5 |
| Peanuts, oil-roasted | 42 | 21.0 | 2.9 | 6.6 | 248 | 0 | 6 |
| Pecans, dried | 42 | 28.8 | 2.3 | 7.2 | 285 | 0 | 0 |

| FOOD DESCRIPTION/PORTION | Wt. (g) | Tot. Fat (g) | Sat. Fat (g) | Poly. Fat (g) | Cal. | Chol. (mg) | Sod. (mg) |
|---|---|---|---|---|---|---|---|
| Pistachio, dry-roasted | 42 | 22.5 | 2.9 | 3.5 | 258 | 0 | 3 |
| Walnuts, Black | 42 | 24.2 | 1.5 | 15.9 | 258 | 0 | 0 |
| Walnuts, English, dried | 42 | 26.4 | 2.4 | 16.7 | 273 | 0 | 5 |

**Seeds (approximately 3 Tbsp.)**

| FOOD DESCRIPTION/PORTION | Wt. (g) | Tot. Fat (g) | Sat. Fat (g) | Poly. Fat (g) | Cal. | Chol. (mg) | Sod. (mg) |
|---|---|---|---|---|---|---|---|
| Pumpkin/Squash, dried | 42 | 19.5 | 3.8 | 8.9 | 231 | 0 | 8 |
| Sesame, roasted and toasted | 42 | 20.4 | 2.9 | 9.0 | 242 | 0 | 5 |
| Sunflower, dried | 42 | 21.2 | 2.3 | 14.0 | 243 | 0 | 2 |

**Salad Dressing**

| FOOD DESCRIPTION/PORTION | Wt. (g) | Tot. Fat (g) | Sat. Fat (g) | Poly. Fat (g) | Cal. | Chol. (mg) | Sod. (mg) |
|---|---|---|---|---|---|---|---|
| Blue Cheese (2 Tbsp.) | 30 | 16.0 | 3.0 | 8.6 | 154 | 0 | 0 |
| French (2 Tbsp.) | 32 | 12.8 | 3.0 | 6.8 | 134 | 0 | 428 |
| Italian (2 Tbsp.) | 30 | 14.2 | 2.0 | 8.2 | 138 | 0 | 232 |
| Mayonnaise (2 Tbsp.) | 28 | 22.0 | 3.2 | 11.4 | 198 | 16 | 156 |
| Mayonnaise-Type (2 Tbsp.) | 30 | 9.8 | 1.4 | 5.2 | 114 | 8 | 208 |
| Sandwich Spread, commercial (2 Tbsp.) | 30 | 10.4 | 1.6 | 6.2 | 120 | 24 | 0 |
| Thousand Island (2 Tbsp.) | 32 | 11.2 | 1.8 | 6.2 | 118 | 10 | 218 |
| Vinegar and Oil (2 Tbsp.) | 32 | 16.0 | 3.0 | 7.8 | 144 | 0 | 0 |

**Other Fats**

| FOOD DESCRIPTION/PORTION | Wt. (g) | Tot. Fat (g) | Sat. Fat (g) | Poly. Fat (g) | Cal. | Chol. (mg) | Sod. (mg) |
|---|---|---|---|---|---|---|---|
| Bacon (see p. 27) | | | | | | | |
| Butter (1 Tbsp.) | 15 | 12.3 | 7.5 | 0.7 | 108 | 33 | 123 |
| Olives, green (5 small) | 17 | 1.8 | 0.2 | 0.2 | 17 | 0 | 343 |
| Olives, ripe (2 extra large) | 14 | 1.7 | 0.2 | 0.2 | 15 | 0 | 97 |
| Peanut Butter, smooth (2 Tbsp.) | 33 | 16.5 | 2.7 | 4.8 | 189 | 0 | 156 |
| Shortening, hydrogenated soybean and cottonseed (1 Tbsp.) | 12 | 12.9 | 3.3 | 3.3 | 114 | 0 | 0 |

| FOOD DESCRIPTION/PORTION | Wt. (g) | Tot. Fat (g) | Sat. Fat (g) | Cal. | Chol. (mg) | Sod. (mg) |
|---|---|---|---|---|---|---|

## BREADS, CEREALS, PASTA, AND STARCHY VEGETABLES

### Breads, Pancakes, Waffles

| FOOD DESCRIPTION/PORTION | Wt. (g) | Tot. Fat (g) | Sat. Fat (g) | Cal. | Chol. (mg) | Sod. (mg) |
|---|---|---|---|---|---|---|
| Bagel, 3″ diameter (1) | 100 | 2.6 | — | 296 | — | 360 |
| Biscuit, made with milk, 2″ diameter (2) | 56 | 5.2 | 1.2 | 182 | — | 544 |
| Bread, rye (2 slices) | 56 | 2.0 | — | 147 | — | 390 |
| Bread, wheat (2 slices) | 56 | 2.3 | — | 143 | — | 302 |
| Bread, white (2 slices) | 46 | 1.8 | 0.4 | 126 | — | 288 |
| Bun, hamburger, 3½″ diameter, or hot dog (1) | 40 | 2.2 | 0.5 | 119 | — | 202 |
| English Muffin, plain (1) | 58 | 1.2 | — | 138 | — | 370 |
| French Toast (2 slices) | 130 | 13.4 | — | 306 | — | 514 |
| Muffin, bran, 2″ diameter bottom (1 large) | 60 | 5.9 | 1.8 | 156 | — | 269 |
| Pancake, with egg, milk, 6″ diameter × ½″ thick (2) | 110 | 8.0 | 2.9 | 246 | — | 618 |
| Popover, 2¾″ top, 2″ bottom, 4″ high in center (2) | 60 | 5.6 | 2.0 | 135 | — | 132 |
| Roll, hard, 3¾″ diameter × 2″ high (1) | 50 | 1.6 | 0.4 | 156 | — | 313 |
| Waffle, 9″ × 9″ × ⅝″ square (1 small) | 112 | 11.0 | 3.5 | 313 | — | 162 |

### Cereals, Ready-to-Eat

| FOOD DESCRIPTION/PORTION | Wt. (g) | Tot. Fat (g) | Sat. Fat (g) | Cal. | Chol. (mg) | Sod. (mg) |
|---|---|---|---|---|---|---|
| 40% Bran Flakes (1 oz.) | 28 | 0.5 | 0 | 93 | 0 | 264 |
| 100% Bran Cereal (1 oz.) | 28 | 0.5 | — | 71 | 0 | 320 |
| Bran Squares (1 oz.) | 28 | 0.8 | — | 91 | 0 | 263 |
| Corn Flakes (1 oz.) | 28 | 0.1 | 0 | 110 | 0 | 351 |
| Crisp Rice, low sodium (1 oz.) | 28 | 0.1 | — | 114 | 0 | 3 |
| Granola, homemade (1 oz.) | 28 | 7.7 | 1.4 | 138 | — | 3 |

| FOOD DESCRIPTION/PORTION | Wt. (g) | Tot. Fat (g) | Sat. Fat (g) | Cal. | Chol. (mg) | Sod. (mg) |
|---|---|---|---|---|---|---|
| Natural Cereal, with raisins and dates (1 oz.) | 28 | 5.2 | 3.5 | 128 | 0 | 12 |
| Puffed Wheat, plain (1 oz.) | 28 | 0.4 | 0 | 104 | 0 | 2 |
| Raisin Bran (1 oz.) | 28 | 0.5 | 0 | 86 | 0 | 202 |
| Shredded Wheat (1 large biscuit) | 24 | 0.3 | 0 | 83 | 0 | 0 |
| Wheat Germ, plain, toasted (1 oz.) | 28 | 3.0 | 0.5 | 108 | 0 | 1 |
| Wheat Nuggets (1 oz.) | 28 | 0.1 | 0 | 101 | 0 | 197 |
| **Cereals, Cooked*** | | | | | | |
| Corn Grits, regular and quick (1 cup) | 242 | 0.5 | 0.1 | 146 | 0 | 0 |
| Farina, regular (1 cup) | 251 | 0.5 | 0 | 134 | 0 | 2 |
| Oat Bran, cooked (1 cup) | 219 | 1.9 | 0.4 | 87 | 0 | 2 |
| Oatmeal, cooked, regular, quick and instant (1 cup) | 234 | 2.4 | 0.4 | 145 | 0 | 1 |
| **Pasta and Rice, Cooked** | | | | | | |
| Macaroni (¾ cup) | 105 | 0.7 | 0.1 | 149 | 0 | 0 |
| Noodles, chow mein (⅔ cup) | 28 | 8.6 | 1.2 | 147 | 0 | 122 |
| Noodles, egg (¾ cup) | 141 | 2.1 | 0.4 | 187 | 47 | 10 |
| Rice, brown (1 cup) | 195 | 1.8 | 0.4 | 216 | 0 | 9 |
| Rice, white (1 cup) | 205 | 0.6 | 0.2 | 264 | 0 | 4 |
| Spaghetti (1 cup) | 140 | 0.9 | 0.1 | 197 | — | 0 |
| **Starchy Vegetables** | | | | | | |
| Corn, Lima Beans, Green Peas, Plantain, White Potato, Winter or Acorn Squash, Yam or Sweet Potato (½ cup) | | 0 | 0 | 80 | 0 | ** |

* Product cooked in unsalted water.
** Canned vegetables are high in sodium unless the label says they are canned without salt.

| FOOD DESCRIPTION/PORTION | Wt. (g) | Tot. Fat (g) | Sat. Fat (g) | Cal. | Chol. (mg) | Sod. (mg) |
|---|---|---|---|---|---|---|
| **Prepared Vegetables** | | | | | | |
| Beans, navy, cooked, boiled | | | | | | |
| (½ cup) | 91 | 0.5 | 0.1 | 129 | 0 | 1 |
| Broadbeans, canned (½ cup) | 128 | 0.3 | 0 | 91 | 0 | 580 |
| Coleslaw/Dressing with | | | | | | |
| table cream (½ cup) | 60 | 1.6 | 0.2 | 42 | 5 | 14 |
| Corn Pudding, whole milk, | | | | | | |
| egg, butter (½ cup) | 125 | 6.6 | 3.2 | 136 | 115 | 69 |
| French Fries, oven-heated, | | | | | | |
| cottage-cut (17) | 84 | 6.9 | 3.2 | 183 | 0 | 39 |
| French Fries, fried in | | | | | | |
| animal and vegetable | | | | | | |
| fat (17) | 84 | 13.9 | 5.7 | 265 | 10 | 181 |
| Lentils, cooked, boiled | | | | | | |
| (½ cup) | 99 | 0.4 | 0.1 | 115 | 0 | 2 |
| Onion Rings, frozen, | | | | | | |
| prepared, heated in | | | | | | |
| oven (7 rings) | 70 | 18.7 | 6.0 | 285 | 0 | 263 |
| Potato, au gratin, with | | | | | | |
| whole milk, butter and | | | | | | |
| cheese (⅔ cup) | 168 | 12.8 | 8.0 | 221 | 40 | 729 |
| Potato, hash brown (½ cup) | 78 | 10.9 | 4.3 | 163 | — | 19 |
| Potato, mashed, with whole | | | | | | |
| milk and margarine | | | | | | |
| (½ cup) | 105 | 4.4 | 1.1 | 111 | 2 | 309 |
| Potato, O'Brien, with whole | | | | | | |
| milk and butter | | | | | | |
| (¾ cup) | 168 | 2.3 | 1.4 | 137 | 7 | 365 |
| Potato, scalloped, with | | | | | | |
| whole milk and butter | | | | | | |
| (⅔ cup) | 167 | 6.2 | 3.8 | 144 | 19 | 560 |
| Potato, Candied Sweet | | | | | | |
| Potatoes, with brown | | | | | | |
| sugar, butter, 2½″ × 2″ | | | | | | |
| piece | 105 | 3.4 | 1.4 | 144 | 8 | 73 |
| Potato Chips (1 oz.) | 28 | 10.1 | 2.6 | 148 | 0 | 133 |

| FOOD DESCRIPTION/PORTION | Wt. (g) | Tot. Fat (g) | Sat. Fat (g) | Cal. | Chol. (mg) | Sod. (mg) |
|---|---|---|---|---|---|---|
| Potato Pancake, with egg, margarine (1) | 76 | 12.6 | 3.4 | 495 | 93 | 388 |
| Potato Puffs, vegetable oil (⅔ cup) | 84 | 9.1 | 4.3 | 186 | 0 | 624 |
| Potato Salad, with egg and mayonnaise (⅔ cup) | 168 | 13.8 | 2.4 | 240 | 115 | 886 |
| Potato Sticks (3 oz.) | 84 | 29.4 | 7.5 | 444 | 0 | 213 |

## Soup

| FOOD DESCRIPTION/PORTION | Wt. (g) | Tot. Fat (g) | Sat. Fat (g) | Cal. | Chol. (mg) | Sod. (mg) |
|---|---|---|---|---|---|---|
| Bean, with bacon, prepared with water (1 cup) | 253 | 5.9 | 1.5 | 173 | 3 | 952 |
| Beef, chunky-style, ready-to-serve (1 cup) | 240 | 5.1 | 2.6 | 171 | 14 | 867 |
| Beef Broth or Bouillon, ready-to-serve (1 cup) | 240 | 0.5 | 0.3 | 16 | tr | 782 |
| Chicken, chunky-style, ready-to-serve (1 cup) | 251 | 6.6 | 2.0 | 178 | 30 | 887 |
| Chicken Broth, prepared with water (1 cup) | 244 | 1.4 | 0.4 | 39 | 1 | 776 |
| Chicken Mushroom, prepared with water (1 cup) | 244 | 9.2 | 2.4 | — | 10 | — |
| Chicken Noodle, prepared with water (1 cup) | 241 | 2.5 | 0.7 | 75 | 7 | 1107 |
| Chicken Rice, prepared with water (1 cup) | 241 | 1.9 | 0.5 | 60 | 7 | 814 |
| Chicken Vegetable, prepared with water (1 cup) | 241 | 2.8 | 0.9 | 74 | 10 | 944 |
| Chili Beef, prepared with water (1 cup) | 250 | 6.6 | 3.3 | 169 | 12 | 1035 |
| Clam Chowder, Manhattan, prepared with water (1 cup) | 244 | 2.3 | 0.4 | 78 | 2 | 1808 |
| Clam Chowder, New England, prepared with milk (1 cup) | 248 | 6.6 | 3.0 | 163 | 22 | 992 |

| FOOD DESCRIPTION/PORTION | Wt. (g) | Tot. Fat (g) | Sat. Fat (g) | Cal. | Chol. (mg) | Sod. (mg) |
|---|---|---|---|---|---|---|
| Cream of Chicken, prepared with water (1 cup) | 244 | 7.4 | 2.1 | 116 | 10 | 986 |
| Cream of Mushroom, prepared with water (1 cup) | 244 | 9.0 | 2.4 | 129 | 2 | 1031 |
| Gazpacho, ready-to-serve (1 cup) | 244 | 2.2 | 0.3 | 57 | 0 | 1183 |
| Minestrone, chunky, ready-to-serve (1 cup) | 240 | 2.8 | 1.5 | 127 | 5 | 864 |
| Minestrone, prepared with water (1 cup) | 241 | 2.5 | 0.5 | 83 | 2 | 911 |
| Oyster Stew, prepared with milk (1 cup) | 245 | 7.9 | 5.1 | 134 | 32 | 1040 |
| Oyster Stew, prepared with water (1 cup) | 241 | 3.8 | 2.5 | 59 | 14 | 980 |
| Split Pea with Ham, prepared with water (1 cup) | 253 | 4.4 | 1.8 | 189 | 8 | 1008 |
| Tomato, prepared with water (1 cup) | 244 | 1.9 | 0.4 | 86 | 0 | 872 |
| Tomato Rice, prepared with water (1 cup) | 247 | 2.7 | 0.5 | 120 | 2 | 815 |
| Vegetarian Vegetable, prepared with water (1 cup) | 241 | 1.9 | 0.3 | 72 | 0 | 823 |

## Crackers

| FOOD DESCRIPTION/PORTION | Wt. (g) | Tot. Fat (g) | Sat. Fat (g) | Cal. | Chol. (mg) | Sod. (mg) |
|---|---|---|---|---|---|---|
| Bread Sticks, 7³⁄₄″ × ³⁄₄″ diameter (5) | 25 | 0.8 | 0.2 | 96 | 0 | 175 |
| Cheese Crackers (5) | 16 | 13.4 | 1.3 | 75 | — | 163 |
| Graham Crackers, 2¹⁄₂″ squares (4) | 28 | 2.6 | 0.6 | 110 | — | 190 |
| Saltines (5 crackers) | 14 | 1.7 | 0.4 | 62 | — | 156 |
| Sandwich-Type, cheese-peanut butter (4 sandwiches) | 28 | 6.8 | 1.8 | 139 | — | 281 |

| FOOD DESCRIPTION/PORTION | Wt. (g) | Tot. Fat (g) | Sat. Fat (g) | Cal. | Chol. (mg) | Sod. (mg) |
|---|---|---|---|---|---|---|
| Teething Crackers (2 pieces) | 14 | 1.4 | 0.6 | 61 | 3 | 33 |

### Baking Ingredients

| FOOD DESCRIPTION/PORTION | Wt. (g) | Tot. Fat (g) | Sat. Fat (g) | Cal. | Chol. (mg) | Sod. (mg) |
|---|---|---|---|---|---|---|
| Cornmeal, dry (1 oz.) | 28 | 0.3 | — | 100 | — | 0 |
| Cornstarch, not packed (1 Tbsp.) | 8 | tr | 0 | 29 | — | 0 |
| Flour, white (1 oz.) | 28 | 0.3 | — | 101 | — | 0 |

## VEGETABLES AND FRUITS

### Vegetables

| FOOD DESCRIPTION/PORTION | Wt. (g) | Tot. Fat (g) | Sat. Fat (g) | Cal. | Chol. (mg) | Sod. (mg) |
|---|---|---|---|---|---|---|
| All vegetables are low in fat and saturated fatty acids ($\frac{1}{2}$ to 1 cup) | | 0.2 | 0 | 25 | 0 | * |
| Asparagus, frozen, cooked (4 spears) | 60 | 0.3 | 0.1 | 17 | 0 | 2 |
| Broccoli, cooked, boiled ($\frac{3}{4}$ cup) | 100 | 0.3 | 0 | 29 | 0 | 11 |
| Garlic, raw (1 clove) | 3 | 0 | 0 | 4 | 0 | 1 |
| Kidney Beans, cooked, boiled ($\frac{1}{2}$ cup) | 100 | 0.6 | 0.1 | 33 | 0 | — |
| Lentils, cooked, stir-fried ($\frac{1}{2}$ cup) | 100 | 0.5 | 0.1 | 101 | 0 | — |
| Lima Beans, frozen, cooked ($\frac{2}{3}$ cup) | 100 | 0.3 | 0.1 | 105 | 0 | 29 |
| Mushrooms, raw ($\frac{1}{2}$ cup pieces) | 35 | 0.2 | 0 | 9 | 0 | 1 |
| Potato, baked, flesh and skin (1 potato) | 202 | 0.2 | 0.1 | 220 | 0 | 16 |
| Potato, boiled, cooked in skin, flesh (1 potato) | 136 | 0.1 | 0 | 119 | 0 | 6 |
| Squash, winter, all varieties, cooked ($\frac{1}{2}$ cup cubed) | 100 | 0.6 | 0.1 | 39 | 0 | 1 |

* Sodium values vary from 2 to 63 mg per $\frac{1}{2}$ cup cooked. Canned vegetables are higher in sodium than fresh or frozen.

| FOOD DESCRIPTION/PORTION | Wt. (g) | Tot. Fat (g) | Sat. Fat (g) | Cal. | Chol. (mg) | Sod. (mg) |
|---|---|---|---|---|---|---|
| Squash, zucchini, cooked, boiled (²/₃ cup) | 100 | 0.1 | 0 | 16 | 0 | 3 |
| Tofu, raw, regular (¹/₄ block) | 116 | 5.6 | 0.8 | 88 | 0 | 8 |

## Fruits

| FOOD DESCRIPTION/PORTION | Wt. (g) | Tot. Fat (g) | Sat. Fat (g) | Cal. | Chol. (mg) | Sod. (mg) |
|---|---|---|---|---|---|---|
| Apple, raw, 2³/₄″ diameter (1) | 138 | 0.5 | 0.1 | 81 | 0 | 1 |
| Applesauce, canned, unsweetened (¹/₂ cup) | 140 | 0.1 | 0 | 61 | 0 | 2 |
| Apricots, medium, raw (4) | 141 | 0.6 | 0 | 68 | 0 | 1 |
| Banana, 9″ long (half) | 57 | 0.3 | 0.1 | 53 | 0 | 1 |
| Blackberries, raw (³/₄ cup) | 108 | 0.4 | 0 | 56 | 0 | 0 |
| Cantaloupe (1 cup cubes) | 160 | 0.4 | 0 | 57 | 0 | 14 |
| Cherries, sweet, raw (12) | 82 | 0.8 | 0.2 | 59 | 0 | 0 |
| Figs, raw (2 medium) | 100 | 0.3 | 0 | 74 | 0 | 2 |
| Fruit Cocktail, canned, juice-packed (¹/₂ cup) | 136 | 0.1 | 0 | 62 | 0 | 4 |
| Grapefruit (half) | 123 | 0.1 | 0 | 37 | 0 | 0 |
| Grapes, raw (15) | 36 | 0.1 | 0 | 23 | 0 | 0 |
| Honeydew Melon (1 cup cubes) | 170 | 0.2 | 0 | 60 | 0 | 17 |
| Kiwifruit (1 large) | 91 | 0.4 | 0 | 55 | 0 | 4 |
| Mango, raw (half) | 104 | 0.3 | 0 | 68 | 0 | 2 |
| Nectarine, 2¹/₂″ diameter (1) | 136 | 0.6 | 0 | 67 | 0 | 0 |
| Orange, 2¹/₂″ diameter (1) | 131 | 0.2 | 0 | 62 | 0 | 0 |
| Papaya (1 cup) | 140 | 0.2 | 0.1 | 54 | 0 | 4 |
| Peach, 2¹/₂″ diameter (1) | 87 | 0.1 | 0 | 37 | 0 | 0 |
| Peaches, canned, water-packed (2 halves) | 154 | 0.1 | 0 | 36 | 0 | 6 |
| Pear, raw (1) | 166 | 0.7 | 0 | 98 | 0 | 1 |
| Pineapple, raw (³/₄ cup) | 116 | 0.5 | 0 | 58 | 0 | 2 |
| Pineapple, canned, juice-packed (¹/₃ cup) | 83 | 0.1 | 0 | 50 | 0 | 1 |
| Plum, raw, 2¹/₈″ diameter (2) | 132 | 0.8 | 0.1 | 72 | 0 | 0 |
| Pomegranate (half) | 77 | 0.2 | 0 | 52 | 0 | 3 |
| Raspberries, raw (1 cup) | 123 | 0.7 | 0 | 61 | 0 | 0 |

| FOOD DESCRIPTION/PORTION | Wt. (g) | Tot. Fat (g) | Sat. Fat (g) | Cal. | Chol. (mg) | Sod. (mg) |
|---|---|---|---|---|---|---|
| Strawberries, raw, whole | | | | | | |
| (1¼ cups) | 186 | 0.7 | 0 | 56 | 0 | 3 |
| Tangerine, 2½″ diameter (2) | 168 | 0.3 | 0 | 74 | 0 | 2 |
| Watermelon (2 cups cubes) | 336 | 1.5 | 0 | 106 | 0 | 7 |
| | | | | | | |
| **Dried Fruits** | | | | | | |
| Apples, uncooked (6 rings) | 42 | 0.2 | 0.2 | 100 | 0 | 36 |
| Apricots, uncooked | | | | | | |
| (12 halves) | 42 | 0.2 | 0 | 97 | 0 | 3 |
| Dates (5) | 42 | 0.2 | 0 | 114 | 0 | 2 |
| Figs, uncooked (2¼) | 42 | 0.5 | 0.2 | 108 | 0 | 5 |
| Prunes, uncooked (5) | 42 | 0.2 | 0 | 101 | 0 | 2 |
| Raisins (¼ cup) | 42 | 0.2 | 0 | 124 | 0 | 4 |
| | | | | | | |
| **Fruit Juices** | | | | | | |
| Apple Juice (6 fluid oz.) | 180 | 0.2 | 0 | 84 | 0 | 6 |
| Cranberry Juice Cocktail | | | | | | |
| (6 fluid oz.) | 176 | 0 | 0 | 103 | 0 | 6 |
| Grape Juice (6 fluid oz.) | 180 | 0.2 | 0 | 111 | 0 | 4 |
| Grapefruit Juice, | | | | | | |
| unsweetened | | | | | | |
| (6 fluid oz.) | 180 | 0.2 | 0 | 68 | 0 | 3 |
| Orange Juice (6 fluid oz.) | 180 | 0.4 | 0 | 79 | 0 | 1 |
| Pineapple Juice (6 fluid oz.) | 180 | 0.1 | 0 | 101 | 0 | 1 |
| Prune Juice (6 fluid oz.) | 180 | 0 | 0 | 127 | 0 | 9 |

## DESSERTS AND SNACKS

### Cakes, Cookies, Pies, and Other Baked Goods

| FOOD DESCRIPTION/PORTION | Wt. (g) | Tot. Fat (g) | Sat. Fat (g) | Cal. | Chol. (mg) | Sod. (mg) |
|---|---|---|---|---|---|---|
| Boston Cream Pie, 2-layer | | | | | | |
| (1/12 of 8″ diameter) | 69 | 6.5 | 2.0 | 208 | — | 128 |
| Brownies, with nuts and | | | | | | |
| icing (1/6 of | | | | | | |
| 7½″ × 5¼″ × 7/8″ pan) | 61 | 10.7 | 4.9 | 246 | 20 | 143 |
| Cake, Angel Food, without | | | | | | |
| frosting (1/12 of 10″ | | | | | | |
| diameter) | 60 | 0.2 | — | 143 | — | 305 |

| FOOD DESCRIPTION/PORTION | Wt. (g) | Tot. Fat (g) | Sat. Fat (g) | Cal. | Chol. (mg) | Sod. (mg) |
|---|---|---|---|---|---|---|
| Cake, Devil's Food, without frosting, 2-layer ($^1/_{16}$ of 9″ diameter) | 56 | 8.7 | 3.4 | 179 | — | 319 |
| Cake, Fruitcake, without frosting ($^1/_{32}$ of 7″ diameter) | 43 | 7.1 | 1.6 | 167 | — | 83 |
| Cake, Pound Cake, without frosting ($^1/_{12}$ of $8^1/_2$″ loaf) | 42 | 12.7 | 7.5 | 204 | 78 | 75 |
| Cake, Sponge Cake, without frosting ($^1/_{12}$ of $9^3/_4$″ diameter) | 66 | 3.8 | 1.2 | 196 | — | 110 |
| Cake, White, without frosting, 2-layer ($^1/_{16}$ of 9″ diameter) | 53 | 7.3 | 2.2 | 163 | — | 218 |
| Cake, Yellow, 2-layer, without frosting ($^1/_{16}$ of 9″ diameter) | 54 | 8.4 | 1.9 | 181 | — | 234 |
| Cake Frosting, chocolate, prepared with milk and fat (3 Tbsp.) | 51 | 7.2 | 3.9 | 195 | — | 33 |
| Cake Frosting, coconut, with boiled frosting (3 Tbsp.) | 30 | 2.4 | 2.1 | 114 | — | 36 |
| Cake Frosting, fudge, made with water (from mix) (3 Tbsp.) | 45 | 3.0 | 0.9 | 156 | — | 108 |
| Cake Frosting, white, boiled (3 Tbsp.) | 18 | 0 | 0 | 57 | — | 24 |
| Cheesecake ($^1/_8$ of 9″ diameter) | 100 | 19.2 | — | 302 | — | 222 |
| Cookies, Chocolate Chip, $2^1/_3$″ diameter (3) | 30 | 8.0 | 2.6 | 139 | 13 | 62 |
| Cookies, Fig Bars (2) | 28 | 1.9 | 0.5 | 106 | — | 90 |
| Cookies, Gingersnaps, 2″ diameter (4) | 28 | 2.5 | 0.6 | 118 | — | 160 |
| Cookies, sandwich, $1^3/_4$″ diameter (3) | 30 | 6.2 | 1.8 | 148 | — | 189 |

| FOOD DESCRIPTION/PORTION | Wt. (g) | Tot. Fat (g) | Sat. Fat (g) | Cal. | Chol. (mg) | Sod. (mg) |
|---|---|---|---|---|---|---|
| Cupcake, plain, no icing, 2½″ diameter (2) | 50 | 7.0 | 1.9 | 182 | — | 150 |
| Cupcake, plain, with white uncooked icing, 2½″ diameter (2) | 70 | 8.2 | 2.7 | 256 | — | 158 |
| Doughnut, cake-type, 3½″ diameter (1) | 25 | 5.8 | 1.2 | 105 | 8 | 139 |
| Doughnut, yeast-type, 3¾″ diameter (1) | 42 | 11.2 | 2.7 | 172 | 8 | 99 |
| Pastry, Danish, 4¼″ diameter × 1″ thick (1) | 65 | 13.6 | 4.5 | 250 | — | 249 |
| Pastry, toaster, commercial (1) | 56 | 6.4 | — | 217 | — | 256 |
| Pie, Apple, 2-crust (⅛ of 9″ diameter) | 118 | 11.9 | 3.4 | 282 | — | 181 |
| Pie, Cherry, 2-crust (⅛ of 9″ diameter) | 118 | 13.3 | 3.5 | 308 | — | 359 |
| Pie, Custard (⅛ of 9″ diameter) | 114 | 12.7 | 4.3 | 249 | — | 327 |
| Pie, Pecan (⅛ of 9″ diameter) | 103 | 23.6 | 3.3 | 431 | — | 228 |
| Pie, Pumpkin (⅛ of 9″ diameter) | 114 | 12.8 | 4.5 | 241 | — | 244 |
| Pie Crust, baked (⅛ of 9″ diameter) | 23 | 7.5 | 1.8 | 113 | — | 138 |

## Candy

| FOOD DESCRIPTION/PORTION | Wt. (g) | Tot. Fat (g) | Sat. Fat (g) | Cal. | Chol. (mg) | Sod. (mg) |
|---|---|---|---|---|---|---|
| Candy Corn (approx. 30 pieces) | 42 | 0.9 | 0.2 | 155 | — | 90 |
| Caramels, plain or chocolate (1½ oz.) | 42 | 4.4 | 2.4 | 170 | — | 96 |
| Chocolate-Coated Peanuts (1½ oz.) | 42 | 17.6 | 4.5 | 239 | — | 26 |
| Fudge, plain (1½ oz.) | 42 | 5.3 | 1.8 | 170 | — | 81 |
| Gumdrops (1½ oz.) | 42 | 0.3 | 0 | 147 | 0 | 15 |
| Hard Candy (1½ oz.) | 42 | 0.5 | 0 | 164 | 0 | 14 |
| Marshmallow (1½ oz.) | 42 | tr | 0 | 135 | 0 | 17 |

| FOOD DESCRIPTION/PORTION | Wt. (g) | Tot. Fat (g) | Sat. Fat (g) | Cal. | Chol. (mg) | Sod. (mg) |
|---|---|---|---|---|---|---|
| Milk Chocolate, plain | | | | | | |
| (1½ oz.) | 42 | 13.8 | 7.7 | 221 | — | 41 |
| Milk Chocolate, almond | | | | | | |
| (1½ oz.) | 42 | 15.2 | 6.8 | 227 | — | 35 |
| Mints, uncoated (1½ oz.) | 42 | 0.9 | 0.2 | 155 | 0 | 90 |

## SAUCES AND GRAVIES

### Dehydrated Sauces

| FOOD DESCRIPTION/PORTION | Wt. (g) | Tot. Fat (g) | Sat. Fat (g) | Cal. | Chol. (mg) | Sod. (mg) |
|---|---|---|---|---|---|---|
| Béarnaise, prepared with milk and butter | | | | | | |
| (½ cup) | 128 | 34.2 | 20.8 | 350 | 94 | 632 |
| Cheese, prepared with milk | | | | | | |
| (½ cup) | 140 | 8.6 | 4.6 | 154 | 26 | 184 |
| Hollandaise, prepared with milk and butter | | | | | | |
| (½ cup) | 128 | 34.2 | 21.0 | 352 | 94 | 568 |
| Mushroom, prepared with water and vinegar | | | | | | |
| (½ cup) | 134 | 5.2 | 2.8 | 114 | 18 | 766 |
| Sour Cream, prepared with milk (½ cup) | 158 | 15.2 | 8.0 | 254 | 46 | 504 |
| Stroganoff, prepared with milk and water (½ cup) | 148 | 5.4 | 3.4 | 136 | 20 | 914 |
| Sweet and Sour, prepared with water and vinegar | | | | | | |
| (½ cup) | 156 | 0 | 0 | 148 | 0 | 390 |
| White, prepared with milk | | | | | | |
| (½ cup) | 132 | 6.8 | 3.2 | 120 | 18 | 398 |

### Ready-to-Serve Sauces

| FOOD DESCRIPTION/PORTION | Wt. (g) | Tot. Fat (g) | Sat. Fat (g) | Cal. | Chol. (mg) | Sod. (mg) |
|---|---|---|---|---|---|---|
| Barbecue (½ Tbsp.) | 16 | 0.3 | 0 | 12 | 0 | 127 |
| Soy (1 Tbsp.) | 18 | 0 | 0 | 11 | 0 | 1029 |
| Teriyaki (1 Tbsp.) | 18 | 0 | 0 | 15 | 0 | 690 |

### Canned Gravies

| FOOD DESCRIPTION/PORTION | Wt. (g) | Tot. Fat (g) | Sat. Fat (g) | Cal. | Chol. (mg) | Sod. (mg) |
|---|---|---|---|---|---|---|
| Au jus (½ cup) | 120 | 0.2 | 0.2 | 20 | 0 | — |

| FOOD DESCRIPTION/PORTION | Wt. (g) | Tot. Fat (g) | Sat. Fat (g) | Cal. | Chol. (mg) | Sod. (mg) |
|---|---|---|---|---|---|---|
| Beef (¹/₂ cup) | 116 | 2.7 | 1.4 | 62 | 4 | 59 |
| Chicken (¹/₂ cup) | 119 | 6.8 | 1.7 | 95 | 3 | 688 |
| Mushroom (¹/₂ cup) | 120 | 3.2 | 0.4 | 60 | 0 | 680 |
| Turkey (¹/₂ cup) | 120 | 2.6 | 0.8 | 62 | 2 | — |

**Dehydrated Gravies**

| FOOD DESCRIPTION/PORTION | Wt. (g) | Tot. Fat (g) | Sat. Fat (g) | Cal. | Chol. (mg) | Sod. (mg) |
|---|---|---|---|---|---|---|
| Au jus, prepared with water (¹/₂ cup) | 124 | 0.4 | 0.2 | 10 | 0 | 290 |
| Brown, prepared with water (¹/₂ cup) | 130 | 0.2 | 0 | 44 | tr | 62 |
| Chicken, prepared with water (¹/₂ cup) | 130 | 1.0 | 0.2 | 42 | 2 | 566 |
| Mushroom, prepared with water (¹/₂ cup) | 128 | 0.4 | 0.2 | 36 | 0 | 702 |
| Onion, prepared with water (¹/₂ cup) | 130 | 0.4 | 0.2 | 40 | 0 | 518 |
| Pork, prepared with water (¹/₂ cup) | 128 | 1.0 | 0.4 | 38 | 2 | 618 |
| Turkey, prepared with water (¹/₂ cup) | 130 | 1.0 | 0.3 | 44 | 2 | 750 |

# Low-Calorie/Low-Fat Menus

*H*ere's a week's worth of menus, all deliciously varied and nutritiously balanced, all low in calories and low in fat. The dishes marked with asterisks are included in the section of low-calorie/low-fat recipes.

# MONDAY

| | | Calories |
|---|---|---:|
| BREAKFAST | Grapefruit Juice (½ cup) | 50 |
| | Small Bagel (1 tsp. margarine, 1 tsp. jam) | 220 |
| | Coffee or Tea | 0 |
| | | 270 |
| LUNCH | Tomato, Cucumber, and Jarlsberg Sandwich (1½ oz. cheese, 1 tsp. margarine, 2 slices pumpernickel) | 375 |
| | Kiwi Fruit (large) | 55 |
| | Skim Milk (1 cup) | 90 |
| | | 520 |
| DINNER | Chicken Teriyaki* | 225 |
| | Baked Potato (2 Tbsp. nonfat yogurt) | 175 |
| | Spinach Salad (1 Tbsp. French Dressing*) | 100 |
| | Sliced Peaches (1 cup, 2 Tbsp. Melba Sauce*) | 125 |
| | Decaffeinated Coffee | 0 |
| | | 625 |

**Total Day's Calories:**    **1,415**

## TUESDAY

|  |  | Calories |
|---|---|---|
| BREAKFAST | Light Cream Cheese (2 oz.) | 120 |
| | Whole-Wheat Toast (2 slices) | 145 |
| | Fresh Pineapple Cubes (1 cup) | 75 |
| | Coffee or Tea | 0 |
| | | 340 |
| LUNCH | Grilled Chicken, Tomato, and Lettuce Sand-wich ($\frac{1}{2}$ skinless breast, 1 tsp. mayon-naise, 2 slices rye) | 350 |
| | Nectarine | 65 |
| | Skim Milk (1 cup) | 90 |
| | | 505 |
| DINNER | Low-Calorie Fillets of Flounder En Papillote* | 190 |
| | Spinach Fettuccine (1 cup) | 200 |
| | Peas ($\frac{1}{2}$ cup) | 65 |
| | Fried Apple Rings* | 140 |
| | Decaffeinated Coffee | 0 |
| | | 595 |

**Total Day's Calories:**  **1,440**

# WEDNESDAY

|  |  | Calories |
|---|---|---:|
| BREAKFAST | High-Fiber Cereal (1 cup, 2 tsp. sugar, ½ cup skim milk) | 225 |
|  | Blueberries (½ cup) | 40 |
|  | Coffee or Tea | 0 |
|  |  | 265 |
| LUNCH | Low-Fat Cheese (two 1-oz. wedges) | 100 |
|  | Small Bagel (1 tsp. margarine) | 200 |
|  | Granny Smith Apple | 80 |
|  | Skim Milk (1 cup) | 90 |
|  |  | 470 |
| DINNER | Brunswick Stew* | 350 |
|  | Spanish Rice* | 195 |
|  | Endive Salad (1 Tbsp. Fresh Herb Dressing*) | 100 |
|  | Strawberries (1 cup, 1 tsp. sugar, 1 Tbsp. nonfat yogurt) | 75 |
|  | Decaffeinated Coffee | 0 |
|  |  | 720 |

**Total Day's Calories:** **1,455**

## THURSDAY

| | | |
|---|---|---:|
| BREAKFAST | Small Bran Muffin | 150 |
| | Cantaloupe Cubes (1 cup) | 60 |
| | Skim Milk (1 cup) | 90 |
| | Coffee or Tea | 0 |
| | | 300 |
| LUNCH | Andalusian Gazpacho* | 150 |
| | Neufchâtel Cream Cheese (1 oz.) | 75 |
| | Large Pita Bread (whole-wheat) | 160 |
| | Small Banana | 65 |
| | | 450 |
| DINNER | Chicken Chow Mein* | 260 |
| | Brown Rice (1 cup) | 215 |
| | Chinese-Style Snow Peas* | 130 |
| | Lichees (1/3 lb.) | 75 |
| | Decaffeinated Coffee | 0 |
| | | 680 |

**Total Day's Calories:**     **1,430**

# FRIDAY

| | | Calories |
|---|---|---|
| BREAKFAST | Nonfat Blueberry Yogurt (1 cup) | 125 |
| | Small Raisin Bagel (1 tsp. margarine) | 200 |
| | Coffee or Tea | 0 |
| | | 325 |
| LUNCH | Turkey Sandwich (3 oz. turkey, lettuce, | |
| | 2 tsp. mayonnaise, 2 slices rye) | 340 |
| | Plum | 35 |
| | Skim Milk (1 cup) | 90 |
| | | 465 |
| DINNER | Flounder à L'Américaine* | 235 |
| | Boiled Potatoes (3 small in jackets) | 150 |
| | Green Beans in Mustard Sauce* | 75 |
| | Lemon Granité* | 135 |
| | White Wine (4 oz.) | 85 |
| | | 680 |

**Total Day's Calories:** **1,470**

## SATURDAY

|  |  | Calories |
|---|---|---|
| BREAKFAST | Granola (⅓ cup) | 185 |
|  | Nonfat Raspberry Yogurt (1 cup) | 125 |
|  | Coffee or Tea | 0 |
|  |  | 310 |
| LUNCH | Russian Salad* | 230 |
|  | Small Pita Bread | 80 |
|  | Skim Milk | 90 |
|  |  | 400 |
| DINNER | Lemony Thai Turkey* | 350 |
|  | Whole-Wheat Linguine (½ cup) | 90 |
|  | Green Salad (1 Tbsp. Buttermilk Dressing*) | 25 |
|  | Poached Meringue Ring* (2 Tbsp. Algarve Apricot Sauce*) | 215 |
|  | White Wine (4 oz.) | 85 |
|  |  | 765 |

**Total Day's Calories:** **1,475**

## SUNDAY

| | | Calories |
|---|---|---:|
| BRUNCH | Rice Pancakes (2 medium, 2 Tbsp. syrup) | 300 |
| | Broiled Canadian Bacon (1 oz.) | 50 |
| | Coffee or Tea | 0 |
| | | 350 |
| LUNCH | Dried Bean Salad* | 215 |
| | Whole-Wheat Bread (1 slice, 1 tsp. margarine) | 105 |
| | Pear | 100 |
| | Skim Milk (1 cup) | 90 |
| | | 510 |
| DINNER | Seafood Provençal* | 220 |
| | Raw Zucchini Salad* | 165 |
| | Small Pita Bread | 80 |
| | Raspberries (1 cup, 2 Tbsp. Low-Calorie Dessert Topping*) | 90 |
| | Decaffeinated Cappuccino | 40 |
| | | 595 |

**Total Day's Calories:** **1,455**

# Low-Calorie/Low-Fat Recipes

*W*hether it's a warming winter soup or some refreshing crab-stuffed pea pods, chicken hash or fruit compote—soup to nuts, a *healthful* recipe need not be a *dull* recipe. Just put fruit in the soup, lemon grass in the turkey, buttermilk in the salad dressing, and then dry-roast your mushrooms till nutty! Select from the following recipes to create your own low-calorie/low-fat menu with a difference.

*Note:* To save space, the following abbreviations are used: NPS *(nutrients per serving)*, NP *(nutrients per* as in *per cookie, per piece, per tablespoon, per teaspoon)*; C *(calorie)*, CH *(cholesterol)*, and S *(sodium)*. Also, g = gram, mg = milligram. If a recipe yields a variable number of servings (4–6, 6–8, etc.), nutritive counts are abbreviated thus: NPS (4–6): 200–135 C, 25–15 mg CH, 40–25 mg S (in each instance the higher number represents 4 servings; the lower, 6). *Note: Unless otherwise indicated, all nutritional counts are based solely upon recipe ingredients and do not include any suggested accompaniments (rice, for example, or potatoes).* Also, whenever recipes call for variable amounts (1–2 tablespoons, $1/4$–$1/2$ cup), the count is figured using the first, or lower, quantity only. Finally, if a recipe suggests alternative ingredients, the calorie count is based upon the principal ingredient, not the alternative.

---

## Tips for Dieters

**Low-Sodium Diets:** Delete salt from recipes (1 tsp. salt = 1,955 mg sodium) or use a salt substitute (1 mg sodium per tsp.); use unsalted butter (1 mg sodium per Tbsp. vs. 116 for the salted) or unsalted margarine (3–4 mg sodium per Tbsp. vs. 87–96 for salted).

**Low-Cholesterol Diets:** Substitute polyunsaturated vegetable oils or margarine (little or no cholesterol) for butter (31 mg cholesterol per Tbsp.) *except in recipes specifying no substitute.*

**Low-Calorie Diets:** Eliminate sugar from savory soups, stews, sauces (1 Tbsp. sugar = 46 calories); use aspartame sweetener (200 times sweeter than sugar, but 4 calories per 1-gram packet) to sweeten ice creams, sherbets, cold fruit desserts, and sauces.

## *APPETIZERS*

### SPINACH, CARROT, AND WHITE KIDNEY BEAN PÂTÉ

**25 servings**

> 2 (10-ounce) packages frozen chopped spinach
> 2 medium-size carrots, peeled and cut in 1″ chunks
> 1 small yellow onion, peeled and quartered
> ¼ pound mushrooms, wiped clean and halved
> ¾ pound zucchini, scrubbed and cut in 1″ chunks
> 2 stalks celery, cut in 1″ chunks

1 (1-pound 3-ounce) can white kidney beans,
     drained
2 eggs, lightly beaten
1 teaspoon salt
$1/4$ teaspoon pepper

Preheat oven to 350° F. Cook spinach by package directions,
dump into a large sieve set over a large heatproof bowl;
press with the back of a spoon to extract as much liquid as
possible. Measure out and reserve $1/4$ cup spinach cooking
liquid. Chop spinach, carrots, onion, and mushrooms very
fine by pulsing in an electric blender at high speed 10–12
times or 6–8 times in a food processor fitted with the metal
chopping blade; dump into a large bowl. Now chop zucchini,
celery, and beans the same way; add to bowl along with all
remaining ingredients. Mix well. Pack into a well-buttered
9″ × 5″ × 3″ baking pan lined on the bottom with buttered
wax paper. Cover with buttered wax paper (buttered-side-
down), set in a large shallow baking pan, pour hot water into
pan to a depth of $1/2$″, and bake, uncovered, $1/4$ hours until
set. Remove wax paper cover and cool pâté in pan, right-
side-up, on a wire rack to room temperature. Unmold carefully on small oblong platter, peel off wax paper, cover, and
chill 3–4 hours. Before serving, let pâté stand about 20 minutes at room temperature.

NPS: 40 C, 20 mg CH, 185 mg S

# CRAB-STUFFED SNOW PEA PODS

**40 stuffed pea pods**

Substitute finely minced cooked shrimp or lobster meat for the crab, if you like. Both are equally delicious.

*40 small snow pea pods, washed and trimmed*
*¹/₂ pound lump crab meat, well picked over, or 1*
    *(6-ounce) can snow crab meat, drained*
*1 hard-cooked egg, peeled*
*¹/₃ cup mayonnaise*
*¹/₄ cup finely chopped celery*
*1 tablespoon minced capers*
*1 teaspoon Dijon mustard*
*¹/₈ teaspoon pepper*

Blanch pea pods in boiling water 10 seconds; drain, plunge into ice water, drain again, and pat dry on paper toweling. Split pea pods open along the straight edge, not quite to the ends, to form "pockets." Mince the crab very fine; mash the egg yolk to a paste and chop the white fine; mix into the crab along with all remaining ingredients. Fill each pea pod with about ³/₄ teaspoon of the crab mixture and flatten slightly. Arrange the pods close together in a shallow dish, cover, and chill 1–2 hours.

NP Pod: 20 C, 10 mg CH, 65 mg S

## ARMENIAN BEAN APPETIZER

4–6 servings

A good addition to antipasto.

*¹/₄ cup olive oil*
*2 tablespoons lemon juice*
*³/₄ teaspoon salt (about)*
*¹/₈ teaspoon white pepper*
*1 clove garlic, peeled and crushed*
*3 tablespoons minced parsley*
*2 cups cooked, drained dried pea beans or navy*
    *beans, flageolets, or cannellini (white kidney*
    *beans)*

Beat oil with lemon juice and salt until creamy, mix in pepper, garlic, and 2 tablespoons parsley. Pour over beans, mix lightly, cover, and marinate 3–4 hours in refrigerator, stirring now and then. Remove from refrigerator, stir well, let stand at room temperature 15–20 minutes, then serve sprinkled with remaining parsley either as a first course in lettuce cups with lemon wedges or spooned onto sesame seed wafers.

NPS (4–6): 235–155 C, 0 mg CH, 420–280 mg S

**VARIATION**

**Turkish Bean Appetizer:** Prepare as directed but add 1 tablespoon minced fresh dill and 1 teaspoon minced fresh mint. Serve topped with paper-thin, raw onion rings. Nutritional count same as basic recipe.

## DRY-ROASTED HERBED MUSHROOMS

**4–6 servings**

An unusual appetizer and oh! so low in calories.

*½ teaspoon garlic salt*
*1 pound medium-size mushrooms, wiped clean and*
*    sliced thin*
*1 teaspoon seasoned salt*
*½ teaspoon oregano*
*½ teaspoon powdered rosemary*

Preheat oven to 200° F. Sprinkle 2 *lightly* oiled baking sheets with garlic salt and arrange mushrooms 1 layer deep on sheets. Mix seasoned salt and herbs and sprinkle evenly over mushrooms. Bake, uncovered, about 1½ hours until dry and crisp but not brown. Cool slightly and serve as a cocktail nibble. (*Note:* Store airtight; these absorb moisture rapidly.)

NPS (4–6): 35–25 C, 0 mg CH, 550–350 mg S

## CAPONATA (SICILIAN EGGPLANT SPREAD)

**3 cups**

Refrigerated, this will keep about a week. Bring to room temperature before serving.

*4 tablespoons olive oil*
*1 small eggplant, cut in 1″ cubes but not peeled*
*1 medium-size yellow onion, peeled and minced*

*1/3 cup minced celery*

*1 cup tomato purée*

*1/3 cup coarsely chopped, pitted green and/or ripe
    olives*

*4 anchovy fillets, minced*

*2 tablespoons capers*

*2 tablespoons red wine vinegar*

*1 tablespoon sugar*

*1/2 teaspoon salt (about)*

*1/4 teaspoon pepper*

*1 tablespoon minced parsley*

Heat 3 tablespoons oil in a large, heavy saucepan 1 minute over moderately high heat, add eggplant and sauté, stirring now and then, 10 minutes until golden and nearly translucent. Add remaining oil, onion, and celery and stir-fry 5–8 minutes until pale golden. Add remaining ingredients except parsley, cover, and simmer 1¼–1½ hours until quite thick, stirring now and then. Mix in parsley, cool to room temperature, taste for salt and adjust as needed. Serve as a spread for crackers.

NP Tablespoon: 20 C, 0 mg CH, 60 mg S

## *SOUPS*

### EASY FISH STOCK

**2 quarts**

Bones of haddock, halibut, cod, sea bass, and/or pike produce a fragrant stock. Use for making seafood soups and sauces.

*2 quarts cold water*
*1 pound fishbones, heads and trimmings*
*1 tablespoon salt*

Place all ingredients in a kettle, cover, and simmer 1 hour. Strain liquid through a fine sieve and use for poaching fish, making soups or sauces. *(Note:* This stock freezes well.)

NP Cup: 5 C, 5 mg CH, 830 mg S

## POTAGE SAINT-GERMAIN

**4 servings**

This soup should be made with fresh young peas, but if they're unavailable, use the frozen. Restaurants sometimes use dried split peas—very good but not authentic.

*2 cups cooked green peas*
*2 cups white stock or a $1/2$ and $1/2$ mixture of water*
*    and beef broth*
*$1/2$ teaspoon minced fresh chervil or $1/4$ teaspoon*
*    dried chervil*
*1 tablespoon butter (no substitute)*
*$1/4$ cup croutons*

Set aside 1 tablespoon peas; put the rest through a food mill or purée by buzzing with a little stock 20–30 seconds in a food processor fitted with the metal chopping blade. Mix purée and stock and strain through a fine sieve, pressing solids to extract as much liquid as possible. Pour into a saucepan, add chervil and butter, and heat, stirring now and then, about 5 minutes until a good serving temperature.

Taste for seasoning and adjust as needed. Stir in reserved peas, ladle into bowls, and sprinkle with croutons.

NPS: 145 C, 10 mg CH, 445 mg S

## QUICK CREAM OF TOMATO SOUP

**6 servings**

> *⅓ cup minced yellow onion*
> *2 tablespoons butter or margarine*
> *2 tablespoons flour*
> *½ teaspoon basil*
> *½ teaspoon oregano*
> *1¼ teaspoons salt*
> *⅛ teaspoon pepper*
> *1 tablespoon tomato paste*
> *1 tablespoon light brown sugar*
> *1 (10½-ounce) can condensed beef consommé*
> *1 cup milk*
> *1 (1-pound 12-ounce) can tomatoes (do not drain)*

Stir-fry onion in butter in a large heavy saucepan 3–5 minutes until limp, blend in flour, herbs, salt, and pepper, then stir in tomato paste, light brown sugar, consommé, and milk and heat, stirring constantly, until thickened and smooth. Put tomatoes through a food mill or purée by churning 15–20 seconds in a food processor fitted with the metal chopping blade; add to pan and simmer, uncovered, 12–15 minutes—do not allow to boil. Ladle into soup bowls and serve piping hot.

NPS: 125 C, 15 mg CH, 970 mg S

# COCKALEEKIE

**4 servings**

This old Scottish cock and leek soup used to be rich as a stew. Today you're more apt to be served the following version—with or without prunes.

> 1 pound leeks, washed, trimmed, halved lengthwise, and sliced $^{1}/_{8}$" thick (include some green tops)
> 1 tablespoon butter or margarine
> 1 quart chicken broth
> $^{1}/_{2}$ teaspoon salt
> $^{1}/_{8}$ teaspoon pepper
> $^{1}/_{2}$ cup diced, cooked chicken meat
> 4–6 whole or coarsely chopped pitted prunes (optional)
> 1 teaspoon minced parsley

Stir-fry leeks in butter in a saucepan over moderately low heat 2–3 minutes. Add all remaining ingredients except parsley, cover, and simmer 10 minutes. Sprinkle with parsley and serve.

NPS: 125 C, 25 mg CH, 1095 mg S
NPS (with prunes): 144 C, 25 mg CH, 1095 mg S

# ARTICHOKE SOUP

**4 servings**

An unusually delicate soup. Good hot or cold.

> 2 *cups globe artichoke hearts (fresh, frozen, or drained canned)*
> 2 *tablespoons butter or margarine*
> 1 *cup milk*
> 2 *cups water*
> 1 *teaspoon salt*
> $\frac{1}{8}$ *teaspoon white pepper*
> 1 *clove garlic, peeled and speared with a toothpick*
> $\frac{1}{2}$ *cup beef consommé*
> 1 *teaspoon minced parsley*

If artichokes are fresh, parboil 20–25 minutes and drain. If frozen, thaw just enough to separate. Quarter hearts, then slice thin crosswise. Stir-fry in butter in a saucepan (not aluminum) over moderately low heat 5 minutes; do not brown. Add all but last 2 ingredients, cover, and simmer over lowest heat 20 minutes. Discard garlic, purée about half the mixture by buzzing 15–20 seconds in a food processor fitted with the metal chopping blade or by putting through a food mill; return to pan. Add consommé and heat to serving temperature, stirring now and then. Serve hot sprinkled with parsley.

NPS: 125 C, 25 mg CH, 760 mg S

**Cold Artichoke Soup:** Slice artichokes but do not fry; omit butter. Simmer as directed, then purée and proceed as above.

NPS: 75 C, 10 mg CH, 700 mg S

## ANDALUSIAN GAZPACHO
## (COLD SPANISH VEGETABLE SOUP)

**6 servings**

Glorious on a hot summer day. And almost a meal in itself.

*³/₄ cup soft white bread crumbs*
*3 tablespoons red wine vinegar*
*2 cloves garlic, peeled and crushed*
*¹/₄ cup olive oil*
*1 large cucumber, peeled, seeded, and cut in fine*
    *dice*
*1 sweet green pepper, cored, seeded, and minced*
*8 large ripe tomatoes, peeled, cored, seeded, and*
    *chopped fine*
*1 cup cold water*
*¹/₂ teaspoon salt*
*¹/₈ teaspoon pepper*

Place bread crumbs, vinegar, garlic, and oil in a small bowl and mix vigorously with a fork to form a smooth paste; set aside. Mix all remaining ingredients in a large mixing bowl, then blend in bread paste. Cover and chill at least 24 hours before serving. Serve icy cold in soup bowls as a first course or as a midafternoon refresher. For a special touch, bed the soup bowls in larger bowls of crushed ice and garnish with sprigs of fresh dill or basil or, failing that, watercress or parsley.

NPS: 150 C, 0 mg CH, 220 mg S

## BASIC FRUIT SOUP

**4 servings**

Slavs and Scandinavians sometimes serve a hot or cold fruit soup before the main course; berries, cherries, and plums are the favored "soup fruits."

> *1 pint berries, washed and stemmed*
> *(strawberries, raspberries, blueberries,*
> *boysenberries, blackberries, or gooseberries)*
> *1 pint water or a ¹/₂ and ¹/₂ mixture of water and*
> *dry white wine*
> *¹/₄ cup sugar (about)*
> *2 teaspoons lemon juice*
> *1 tablespoon cornstarch blended with 2*
> *tablespoons cold water*

Simmer berries in water in a covered saucepan 10 minutes until mushy; purée by buzzing 15–20 seconds in an electric blender at low speed or 10–15 seconds in a food processor fitted with the metal chopping blade; press through a fine sieve. Return purée to pan, add remaining ingredients, and heat to a boil, stirring. Taste for sugar and add more, if needed. Serve hot or cold.

NPS (with water only): 80 C, 0 mg CH, 1 mg S
NPS (with strawberries & wine): 90 C, 0 mg CH, 5 mg S
NPS (with blueberries & wine): 105 C, 0 mg CH, 10 mg S

**Quick Berry Soup:** Substitute 2 (10-ounce) packages thawed frozen berries or 1 (1-pound) undrained can berries for the fresh. Do not cook; purée and sieve, then add enough water to make 1 quart. Heat with sugar (just enough to taste), lemon juice, and cornstarch paste as directed. Nutritional count about the same as basic recipe.

**Spiced Fruit Soup:** Prepare as directed, adding ½ teaspoon cinnamon and ¼ teaspoon each nutmeg and cloves along with sugar. Nutritional count about the same as basic recipe.

**Sweet-Sour Fruit Soup:** Prepare as directed, increasing sugar to 5 tablespoons and adding, at the same time, 3 tablespoons red or white wine vinegar.

NPS: 90 C, 0 mg CH, 5 mg S

**Plum Soup:** Substitute 1 pound purple plums for berries and simmer 25–30 minutes until mushy; cool slightly, pit, then purée and proceed as for Basic Fruit Soup.

NPS: 115 C, 0 mg CH, 1 mg S

## APPLE SOUP

**4–6 servings**

Serve as a first course or light dessert.

*1 pound greenings or other tart cooking apples,*
*    peeled, cored, and sliced thin*
*3 cups water*

*1 teaspoon grated lemon rind*
*2 teaspoons lemon juice*
*¹/₂ cup sugar (about)*
*¹/₂ teaspoon cinnamon*
*¹/₄ teaspoon nutmeg*

Place ingredients in a saucepan, cover, and simmer about 20 minutes until apples are mushy. Purée by buzzing 15–20 seconds in an electric blender at low speed or 10–15 seconds in a food processor fitted with the metal chopping blade; taste for sugar and add more if needed. Serve hot or cold.

NPS (4–6): 155–100 C, 0 mg CH, 1 mg S

VARIATION
**Russian Apple Soup:** Prepare as directed, using 2 cups water and 1 cup red Bordeaux wine for cooking the apples. Before puréeing, add ¹/₄ cup red or black currant jelly and stir until melted. Purée and serve hot or cold.

NPS (4–6): 215–145 C, 0 mg CH, 5 mg S

## *POULTRY*

### CHICKEN TERIYAKI

**6 servings**

*3 large boneless chicken breasts, halved and*
*skinned*
*¹/₂ cup soy sauce*
*¹/₄ cup mirin (sweet rice wine) or medium or dry*
*sherry*

*1 tablespoon sugar*
*2 teaspoons finely grated fresh gingerroot*

Place chicken breasts between wax paper and pound to flatten slightly. Marinate 1–2 hours in refrigerator in a mixture of soy sauce, *mirin,* sugar, and ginger, turning once or twice. Preheat broiler. Remove chicken from marinade and arrange on lightly oiled rack in broiler pan. Broil 5″–6″ from heat about 4 minutes on each side; brush with marinade when turning. Serve with tiny bowls of remaining marinade (sake cups are a good size) or pour a little marinade over each portion. Good with boiled rice and a spinach salad.

NPS: 225 C, 100 mg CH, 1880 mg S

## CHICKEN CHOW MEIN

**6 servings**

*$^1/_2$ pound mushrooms, wiped clean and sliced thin*
*6 scallions, minced (include some tops)*
*2 small sweet green peppers, cored, seeded, and*
    *minced*
*4 stalks celery, minced*
*2 tablespoons cooking oil*
*$2^1/_2$ cups chicken broth*
*2 tablespoons soy sauce*
*$^1/_4$ cup cornstarch blended with $^1/_4$ cup cold water*
*$^1/_2$ teaspoon salt*
*$^1/_8$ teaspoon pepper*
*3 cups bite-size pieces cooked chicken meat,*
    *preferably white meat*
*1 pound bean sprouts, washed*

1 (4-ounce) can water chestnuts, drained and
    sliced thin

Stir-fry mushrooms, scallions, green peppers, and celery in
oil in a large, heavy skillet over moderately high heat 8–10
minutes until golden brown. Add broth and soy sauce, turn
heat to low, cover, and simmer 10 minutes. Mix in cornstarch paste, salt, and pepper and heat, stirring constantly,
until thickened and clear. Add chicken, bean sprouts, and
water chestnuts and heat and stir about 5 minutes, just to
heat through. Taste for salt and adjust if needed. Serve over
boiled rice.

NPS: 260 C, 60 mg CH, 1055 mg S


## MOO GOO GAI PEEN (CHICKEN WITH MUSHROOMS)

**2 servings**

   1 large boneless chicken breast, halved and
       skinned
   2 tablespoons peanut oil
   $1/2$ cup thinly sliced mushrooms
   1 cup finely shredded Chinese cabbage
   $1/3$ cup thinly sliced bamboo shoots
   2 ($1/2$") cubes fresh gingerroot, peeled and crushed
   $1/3$ cup chicken broth
   1 tablespoon dry sherry (optional)
   $1/4$ pound snow pea pods, washed and trimmed
   3 water chestnuts, sliced thin
   2 teaspoons cornstarch blended with 1 tablespoon
       cold water
   $3/4$ teaspoon salt (about)
   $1/8$ teaspoon sugar

Cut chicken across the grain into strips about 2″ long and ¼″ wide; set aside. Heat 1 tablespoon oil in a large, heavy skillet over moderately high heat about 1 minute, add mushrooms, cabbage, bamboo shoots, and ginger, and stir-fry 2 minutes. Add broth, cover, and simmer 2–3 minutes. Pour all into a bowl and set aside. Wipe out skillet, heat remaining oil, and stir-fry chicken 2–3 minutes; if you like sprinkle with sherry and stir a few seconds longer. Return vegetables and broth to skillet, add snow peas and chestnuts, and heat, stirring until bubbling. Mix in cornstarch paste, salt, and sugar and heat, stirring until clear and slightly thickened; taste for salt and adjust as needed. Serve with boiled rice.

NPS: 380 C, 100 mg CH, 1080 mg S

### BRUNSWICK STEW

**12–15 servings**

American Indian women, who invented Brunswick Stew, used to make it with squirrel or rabbit. If you have a hunter in the family, try it their way.

> 1 (6-pound) stewing hen or capon, cleaned and
>     dressed
> 1 gallon cold water
> 2 stalks celery (include tops)
> 1 tablespoon sugar
> 5 medium-size potatoes, peeled and cut in ½″
>     cubes
> 3 medium-size yellow onions, peeled and coarsely
>     chopped
> 6 large ripe tomatoes, peeled, cored, seeded, and
>     coarsely chopped

2 (10-ounce) packages frozen baby lima beans (do
    not thaw)
2 (10-ounce) packages frozen whole kernel corn (do
    not thaw)
1 medium-size sweet green pepper, cored and cut
    in short, thin slivers
2 tablespoons salt (about)
$^1/_4$ teaspoon pepper

Remove fat from body cavity of bird, then place bird and
giblets in a very large kettle. Add water and celery, cover,
and simmer 1–2 hours until *just* tender. Remove bird and
giblets from broth and cool. Strain broth and skim off fat.
Rinse kettle, pour in broth, add sugar, all vegetables but
corn and green pepper, cover, and simmer 1 hour. Meanwhile, skin chicken, cut meat in 1″ chunks and dice giblets.
Return chicken and giblets to kettle, add remaining ingredients, cover, and simmer 40–45 minutes, stirring occasionally.
Taste for salt, adding more if needed. Serve piping hot in
soup bowls as a main dish.

NPS (12–15): 350–280 C, 90–70 mg CH, 1250–1000 mg S

### CHICKEN OR TURKEY HASH

**4 servings**

1 medium-size yellow onion, peeled and minced
$^1/_2$ medium-size sweet green or red pepper, cored,
    seeded, and minced (optional)
2 tablespoons bacon drippings, butter, or
    margarine
2 cups diced cooked chicken or turkey meat

2 *cups diced cooked cold peeled potatoes, sweet*
   *potatoes, or yams*
1/4 *cup applesauce*
1 *tablespoon minced parsley*
1 *teaspoon salt*
1/8 *teaspoon pepper*
1/2 *teaspoon poultry seasoning*

Stir-fry onion and, if you like, green pepper in drippings in a large, heavy skillet over moderate heat 5–8 minutes until onion is pale golden. Mix in all remaining ingredients, pat down with a broad spatula, and cook, uncovered, without stirring about 10 minutes until a brown crust forms on the bottom. Using 2 broad spatulas, turn hash and brown flip side 8–10 minutes. Cut into 4 portions and serve.

NPS (Chicken): 250 C, 65 mg CH, 650 mg S
NPS (Turkey): 240 C, 60 mg CH, 640 mg S

## LEMONY THAI TURKEY WITH SHIITAKE MUSHROOMS AND BEAN SPROUTS

### 4 servings

This recipe is "medium hot." If you like really torrid food, as many Thais do, increase amount of chili peppers to suit.

1 *pound turkey cutlets, cut* 1/4" *thick and pounded*
   *thin as for scaloppine*
4 *tablespoons peanut oil*
2 *cloves garlic, peeled and minced*
2 (1/2") *cubes fresh gingerroot, peeled and minced*
1/8–1/4 *teaspoon crushed dried hot red chili peppers*

*1 teaspoon minced lemon grass or finely grated lemon rind*

*1 bunch scallions, washed, trimmed, and coarsely chopped (include some tops)*

*¹/₄ pound shiitake mushrooms, rinsed, dried, and coarsely chopped, or ¹/₂ cup dried Chinese black mushrooms, prepared for cooking and coarsely chopped*

*1 pound bean sprouts, washed*

*2 tablespoons dark brown sugar*

*¹/₄ cup soy sauce*

*2 tablespoons chicken broth, water, or dried mushroom soaking liquid*

Cut turkey cutlets across the grain into strips 2″ long and ¹/₄″ wide. Stir-fry turkey in 2 tablespoons oil in a large heavy skillet or wok set over moderately high heat 2–3 minutes; remove and reserve. With a mortar and pestle, pound garlic with gingerroot, chilies, and lemon grass until well bruised; set aside. Heat remaining oil in skillet, add scallions, mushrooms, and garlic mixture and stir-fry 2 minutes. Add ³/₄ of bean sprouts and stir-fry 2 minutes longer. Reduce heat to moderate; combine brown sugar, soy sauce, and chicken broth and pour over vegetables; add turkey, mix well, then cook and stir 2 minutes until steaming hot. Serve at once sprinkled with remaining raw bean sprouts. Accompany with boiled rice.

NPS: 350 C, 70 mg CH, 1440 mg S

## SOLE OR FLOUNDER À L'AMÉRICAINE

**6 servings**

2 pounds sole or flounder fillets
1 teaspoon salt
1/8 teaspoon white pepper
1 cup dry white wine
1 cup boiling water

SAUCE AMÉRICAINE
1 small yellow onion, peeled and minced
1 carrot, peeled and cut in small dice
3 tablespoons minced shallots or scallions
1 clove garlic, peeled and crushed
2 tablespoons cooking oil
1/4 cup brandy
2 large tomatoes, peeled, cored, seeded, and
    coarsely chopped
2 tablespoons tomato paste
1 cup Easy Fish Stock
1 cup dry white wine
1 teaspoon tarragon
1 teaspoon minced parsley
1 (6–8 ounce) frozen rock lobster tail
1 tablespoon butter or margarine
1/4 teaspoon sugar
Pinch cayenne pepper

Prepare sauce early in the day to allow flavors to blend: Sauté onion, carrot, shallots, and garlic in oil in a saucepan over moderate heat 3–5 minutes until onion is very pale golden. Add brandy, warm briefly, remove from heat, and blaze with a match. Add all but last 3 sauce ingredients, cover, and simmer 10 minutes; remove lobster, take meat from shell, slice crosswise 1/4″ thick, and refrigerate. Continue simmering sauce, *uncovered,* about 1 hour, stirring occasionally. Liquid should be reduced by half; if not, boil rapidly to reduce. Strain liquid through a fine sieve into a small saucepan, pressing vegetables lightly. Heat 1–2 minutes over low heat, whisk in butter, sugar, and cayenne, taste for salt and adjust as needed. Cover and set aside. About 10 minutes before serving, fold fillets envelope fashion, ends toward middle, and arrange in a large skillet (not iron); sprinkle with salt and pepper. Pour in wine and water, cover and simmer slowly 7–10 minutes until fish will just flake. Meanwhile, add lobster to sauce and reheat slowly until bubbly. Using a slotted spoon, lift fish to a hot deep platter, smother with sauce, and serve.

NPS: 235 C, 95 mg CH, 730 mg S

## LOW-CALORIE FILLETS OF
## FLOUNDER EN PAPILLOTE

**4 servings**

*4 large flounder fillets (about 1½ pounds)*
*1½ teaspoons salt*
*½ cup minced scallions*
*1 tablespoon butter or margarine*
*1 tablespoon flour*

2 ripe tomatoes, peeled, cored, seeded, and
    chopped fine
1 teaspoon red or white wine vinegar
$^{1}/_{2}$ teaspoon basil or oregano
$^{1}/_{8}$ teaspoon pepper

Preheat oven to 350° F. Cut 4 large squares of cooking
parchment (available at specialty food shops) or heavy duty
foil (large enough to wrap fillets); lay a fillet on each and
sprinkle with 1 teaspoon salt. Sauté scallions in butter in a
small skillet over moderate heat 3–5 minutes until limp;
sprinkle in flour, add remaining salt and all other ingredients, and heat, stirring, over low heat 3–5 minutes to blend
flavors. Spoon a little sauce over each fillet and wrap tightly
drugstore style. Place packages on a baking sheet and bake
30–40 minutes; unwrap 1 package and check to see if fish
flakes; if not, rewrap and bake a little longer. Serve in foil to
retain all juices.

NPS: 190 C, 90 mg CH, 990 mg S

## SEAFOOD PROVENÇAL

**6 servings**

2 pounds fillets or steaks of delicate white fish (cod,
    haddock, flounder, fluke, halibut, etc.)
$1^{1}/_{2}$ teaspoons salt
$^{1}/_{4}$ teaspoon pepper
1 clove garlic, peeled and crushed
1 cup Easy Fish Stock
3 firm tomatoes, halved but not peeled
2 tablespoons olive or other cooking oil
$^{1}/_{8}$ teaspoon thyme

*¹/₂ cup soft white bread crumbs*
*2 tablespoons melted butter or margarine*

Preheat oven to 350° F. Fold fillets envelope fashion, ends toward center, and arrange in a single layer in a well-buttered shallow 2¹/₂-quart casserole. Sprinkle with 1 teaspoon salt and ¹/₈ teaspoon pepper. Stir garlic into stock and pour over fish. Bake, uncovered, basting two or three times, 20–30 minutes until fish will flake. Meanwhile, sauté tomatoes in oil in a skillet over moderate heat 4–5 minutes until lightly browned; keep warm. When fish is done, draw liquid off with a bulb baster. Arrange tomatoes around fish, sprinkle with thyme and remaining salt and pepper. Top with crumbs, drizzle with butter, and broil 3″–4″ from heat 1–2 minutes to brown.

NPS: 220 C, 85 mg CH, 850 mg S


### SASHIMI (JAPANESE-STYLE RAW FISH AND VEGETABLES)

**6 main course servings, enough appetizers for 10**

Prepare as the Japanese do, paying great attention to the artistic arrangement of fish and garnishes on small colored plates. Serve as an appetizer or main course with *sake.*

*2 pounds fresh pompano, red snapper, or tuna*
   *fillets*
*1 cucumber, sliced paper thin (do not peel)*
*Watercress sprigs*

CONDIMENTS
*Soy sauce*
*$^1/_2$ cup minced white radishes*
*$^1/_3$ cup minced fresh gingerroot*
*$^1/_4$ cup prepared horseradish*
*Powdered mustard*
Mirin *or dry sherry*

Insist that the fish is *ocean*-fresh; chill well, then with an extra-sharp knife, slice $^1/_8''$ thick across the grain and slightly on the bias. Cut slices into strips about $1'' \times 2''$ and arrange slightly overlapping on 6 individual plates. Cover and chill until near serving time.

*Setting Up the Sashimi:* At each place set out a small bowl of soy sauce and, in the center of the table, group colorful bowls of minced radishes, gingerroot, horseradish, and mustard, each with its own spoon, around a bottle of *mirin* or sherry.

*Serving the Sashimi:* Arrange cucumber slices and watercress sprigs on plates with raw fish and set on larger plates filled with crushed ice.

*Eating Sashimi:* Before anyone eats anything, he or she mixes a dip by adding a little of the condiments in the center of the table to his bowl of soy sauce. The procedure is then simply to pick up slices of raw fish or cucumber, one at a time, with chopsticks or fork, dip in sauce, and eat.

NPS (6–10) (without condiments): 265–160 C, 85–50 mg CH, 85–50 mg S

**Scallops Sashimi:** Instead of using thin slices of raw fish, substitute 2 pounds tiny whole raw bay scallops, well washed and chilled.

NPS (6–10) (without condiments): 135–80 C, 50–30 mg CH, 400–240 mg S

## *RICE AND VEGETABLES*

### SPANISH RICE

**4 servings**

> 1 large yellow onion, peeled and minced
> 2 tablespoons cooking oil
> 1 small sweet green pepper, cored, seeded, and
>        minced
> $^1/_2$ cup uncooked rice
> $^1/_4$ teaspoon chili powder
> 1 (1-pound) can tomatoes (do not drain)
> $^1/_2$ cup water
> 1 bay leaf, crumbled
> $^3/_4$ teaspoon salt
> $^1/_8$ teaspoon pepper
> $^1/_4$ teaspoon sugar

Sauté onion in oil in a heavy saucepan over moderate heat 5–8 minutes until limp. Add green pepper and stir-fry 5 minutes. Stir in rice and chili powder and brown rice lightly. Add remaining ingredients, chopping up tomatoes, cover, and simmer 20 minutes. Uncover and cook 5 minutes longer.

NPS: 195 C, 0 mg CH, 570 mg S

## KHICHIRI (EAST INDIAN RICE AND LENTILS)

**4–6 servings**

Good topped with yogurt or chutney and especially good with curry.

> *¹/₂ cup dried lentils, washed and sorted*
> *1 medium-size yellow onion, peeled and minced*
> *2¹/₂ cups chicken broth or water*
> *¹/₂ cup uncooked rice*
> *³/₄ teaspoon salt (about)*
> *Pinch crushed dried hot red chili peppers*
> *2 tablespoons margarine*
> *2 teaspoons cumin seeds*

Simmer lentils and onion in broth in a covered heavy saucepan 25 minutes, stirring occasionally. Add rice, salt, and chili peppers, cover, and simmer 20 minutes until rice is tender and all liquid absorbed. Uncover and cook 2–3 minutes to dry out. Meanwhile, melt margarine in a small skillet over moderately low heat, add cumin seeds, and stir-fry ¹/₂ minute until they begin to pop. Pour over rice and toss with a fork. Taste for salt and adjust as needed.

NPS (4–6) (with chicken broth): 255–170 C, 0 mg CH, 975–650 mg S

## ARTICHOKE BOTTOMS STUFFED WITH VEGETABLES

**4 servings**

> *8 globe artichoke hearts, boiled and drained*
> *¼ cup butter or margarine*
> *1½ cups hot seasoned vegetables (asparagus tips or cauliflowerets; chopped spinach; peas and diced carrots; or sautéed chopped mushrooms)*
> *2 tablespoons minced parsley*

Strip all leaves from the hearts and remove chokes. Melt butter in a large skillet over moderately low heat and sauté bottoms 3–4 minutes, basting all the while. Fill with vegetables and sprinkle with parsley.

NPS (asparagus): 150 C, 30 mg CH, 160 mg S
NPS (spinach): 150 C, 30 mg CH, 190 mg S
NPS (peas and carrots): 165 C, 30 mg CH, 210 mg S
NPS (mushrooms): 200 C, 45 mg CH, 215 mg S

**VARIATIONS**

All variations too flexible for meaningful nutritional counts.

**To Serve Cold:** Instead of sautéing bottoms in butter, marinate 2–3 hours in the refrigerator in French Dressing. Fill with cold, seasoned, cooked vegetables.

**Artichoke Bottoms Princesse:** Fill with puréed, cooked, seasoned green peas.

# CHINESE ASPARAGUS

**4–6 servings**

> 2 *pounds asparagus, prepared for cooking*
> 1 *tablespoon cornstarch*
> 2 *tablespoons cold water*
> 1 *cup chicken broth*
> 2 *teaspoons soy sauce*
> 1 *tablespoon dry sherry*
> 1/4 *teaspoon sugar*
> 3 *tablespoons peanut or other vegetable oil*
> 1/4 *cup thinly sliced water chestnuts or bamboo*
>      *shoots*

Cut each asparagus stalk diagonally into slices 1/4" thick. Blend cornstarch with water in a small saucepan, add broth, soy sauce, sherry, and sugar, and heat, stirring, over moderate heat until slightly thickened. Remove from burner but keep warm. Heat oil in a large, heavy skillet or *wok* over moderate heat 1 minute. Add asparagus and stir-fry 3 minutes until crisp-tender. Slowly stir in sauce and heat 2 minutes longer, stirring constantly. Add water chestnuts or bamboo shoots and serve.

NPS (4–6): 115–75 C, 0 mg CH, 415–280 mg S

## GREEN BEANS IN MUSTARD SAUCE

**4 servings**

*1 pound green beans, boiled and drained (reserve*
*cooking water)*
*1 tablespoon butter or margarine*
*1 tablespoon flour*
*Green bean cooking water + enough milk to total ³/₄*
*cup*
*3 tablespoons prepared mild yellow mustard*
*1 tablespoon Worcestershire sauce*
*¹/₂ teaspoon salt*
*¹/₄ teaspoon cayenne pepper*

Keep beans warm. Melt butter over moderate heat and blend in flour. Add the ³/₄ cup liquid and heat, stirring constantly, until thickened. Mix in remaining ingredients and heat, stirring, 2–3 minutes to blend flavors. Pour sauce over beans, toss lightly to mix, and serve.

NPS: 75 C, 10 mg CH, 495 mg S

# HOT MACÉDOINE OF VEGETABLES

**4–6 servings**

A macédoine of vegetables is a mixture of cooked vegetables of similar size and shape. Usually they're diced, sometimes cut in diamonds or small balls. Almost any mixture can be used if the colors and flavors go well together (avoid using beets because their color runs).

*1 cup diced cooked carrots*
*1 cup diced cooked turnips*
*1 cup diced cooked celery*
*1 cup cooked green peas*
*1 cup cooked baby limas*
*1 cup cooked green or wax beans, cut in ¹/₂″ lengths*
*3–4 tablespoons butter or margarine*
*Salt*
*Pepper*

Drain all vegetables well and place in a saucepan with butter and salt and pepper to taste. Warm over low heat 2–3 minutes, shaking pan, until butter melts and serve.

NPS (4–6): 200–135 C, 25–15 mg CH, 280–185 mg S

**VARIATION**

**Cold Macédoine of Vegetables:** Chill cooked vegetables in ice water, drain, pat dry on paper toweling, and refrigerate until ready to use. Instead of seasoning with butter, salt, and pepper, dress with vinaigrette dressing or thin mayonnaise. Serve as a salad, cold vegetable, or hors d'oeuvre. NPS (4–6): 220–145 C, 20–10 mg CH, 250–165 mg S

## CUCUMBERS PROVENÇAL

**4 servings**

> 3 *medium-size cucumbers, peeled, seeded, cut in 1″*
> *cubes, parboiled, and drained*
> 2 *tablespoons butter or margarine*
> 2 *tablespoons olive or other cooking oil*
> 1 *clove garlic, peeled and crushed*
> 2 *medium-size ripe tomatoes, peeled, seeded, and*
> *coarsely chopped*
> 1 *tablespoon minced parsley*
> $^1/_2$ *teaspoon salt*
> $^1/_8$ *teaspoon pepper*

Pat cucumbers dry on paper toweling. Melt butter in a large, heavy skillet over moderate heat, add oil and heat $^1/_2$ minute. Sauté garlic $^1/_2$ minute until pale golden, add cucumbers and tomatoes, and sauté 4–5 minutes until tender, stirring constantly. Off heat, add remaining ingredients, toss lightly to mix, and serve.

NPS: 150 C, 15 mg CH, 345 mg S

## PISTO (SPANISH VEGETABLE STEW)

**16 vegetable servings, appetizers for 50**

*Pisto,* Spanish cousin to *ratatouille,* can be eaten hot or cold, as an appetizer, vegetable, or main dish, depending on how much meat goes into it.

> *1 cup diced lean cooked ham*
> *¹/₂ cup olive oil*
> *4 large yellow onions, peeled and sliced thin*
> *2 medium-size sweet red peppers, cored, seeded, and coarsely chopped*
> *1 (7-ounce) can pimientos, drained and cut in ¹/₄″ strips*
> *4 cloves garlic, peeled and crushed*
> *1 medium-size eggplant, washed and cut in ¹/₂″ cubes (do not peel)*
> *¹/₂ pound mushrooms, wiped clean and sliced thin*
> *2–3 teaspoons salt*
> *2 (9-ounce) packages frozen artichoke hearts (do not thaw)*
> *2 (1-pound) cans tomatoes (do not drain)*

Brown ham in the oil in a large kettle over moderate heat. Add onions, peppers, pimientos, garlic, eggplant, and mushrooms, cover, and simmer slowly, stirring occasionally, 15 minutes until onions are golden. Add remaining ingredients and simmer, covered, 30–40 minutes until artichokes are tender. Cool, cover, and chill 4–5 hours.

NPS (16–50): 130–40 C, 5–1 mg CH, 480–155 mg S

## CHINESE-STYLE SNOW PEAS

**4–6 servings**

*1 pound small snow pea pods, prepared for cooking*
*1 small yellow onion, peeled and minced*
*1 clove garlic, peeled and minced*
*1 (1″) cube fresh gingerroot, peeled and minced*
*2 tablespoons peanut or sesame oil*
*2 tablespoons hot water*
*1–2 tablespoons soy sauce*

Pat snow peas dry on paper toweling. Stir-fry onion, garlic, and gingerroot in oil in a large heavy skillet or *wok* over moderately high heat 1–2 minutes until limp. Add snow peas and water, reduce heat to moderate, cover and cook *1 minute.* Remove lid and cook, stirring constantly, until water evaporates. Mix in soy sauce and serve.

NPS (4–6): 130–85 C, 0 mg CH, 335–225 mg S

**VARIATIONS**

**Chinese-Style Broccoli Flowerets:** For the snow peas, substitute 1 (2-pound) head broccoli, divided into small flowerets. Proceed as recipe directs, allowing broccoli to cook 3–4 minutes.

NPS (4–6): 105–70 C, 0 mg CH, 370–245 mg S

**Chinese-Style Asparagus Tips:** For the snow peas, substitute 2 pounds asparagus, prepared for cooking (use tips only, save stalks for soup). Proceed as recipe directs, allowing asparagus to cook 2 minutes.

NPS (4–6): 75–50 C, 0 mg CH, 335–220 mg S

## STEWED TOMATOES

**4 servings**

Another basic recipe that invites improvisation.

> *4 large ripe tomatoes, peeled, cored, and*
> *quartered, or 1¹/₂ pounds Italian plum*
> *tomatoes, peeled*
> *1 tablespoon water (optional)*
> *³/₄ teaspoon salt*
> *¹/₄ teaspoon sugar*
> *Pinch pepper*

Place tomatoes in a heavy saucepan, add water (if they seem dry) and remaining ingredients. Cover and simmer 5–7 minutes until *just* soft; uncover and simmer ¹/₂ minute longer. Serve in small bowls as a vegetable.

NPS: 35 C, 0 mg CH, 415 mg S

VARIATIONS

**Savory Stewed Tomatoes:** Cook any of the following with the tomatoes: 2 tablespoons minced yellow onion or scallions and ¹/₂ crushed clove garlic; ¹/₄ cup minced celery or sweet green pepper; 1 bay leaf; 1 teaspoon minced fresh basil, oregano, or marjoram, or ½ teaspoon of the dried.

NPS: 35 C, 0 mg CH, 5 mg S

**Stewed Vegetables:** Just before serving, stir in any of the following: 1 cup hot cooked whole kernel corn; 1 cup sautéed sliced mushrooms; 1½ cups hot cooked green beans; 2 cups hot cooked baby okra pods. Recipe too flexible for a meaningful nutritional count.


*SALADS*


### WINTER HEALTH SALAD

**4–6 servings**

A brilliant combination of vegetables.

> *2 cups finely shredded cabbage*
> *1 sweet green pepper, cored, seeded, and cut in julienne strips*
> *1 pimiento, seeded and cut in julienne strips*
> *1 medium-size carrot, coarsely grated (scrub but do not peel)*
> *1 small red onion, peeled and minced, or ¼ cup minced scallions (include tops)*
> *½ cup minced celery (include tops)*
> *½ cup minced cucumber (do not peel unless cucumbers are waxed)*
> *½ small white turnip, peeled and finely grated*
> *⅓ cup tiny cauliflowerets or broccoli flowerets (optional)*

*4 radishes, thinly sliced*
*¹/₄–¹/₃ cup French Dressing*

Chill all vegetables well; add just enough dressing to coat all lightly, toss, and serve.

NPS (4–6) (with cauliflower): 130–90 C, 0 mg CH, 85–55 mg S

VARIATION
**Extra-Low-Calorie Winter Health Salad:** Prepare as directed but dress with Tangy Low-Calorie Salad Dressing.

NPS (4–6) (with cauliflower): 65–40 C, 0 mg CH, 165–110 mg S

## RAW ZUCCHINI SALAD

**4–6 servings**

Use only the tenderest young zucchini for making this salad. Otherwise it may be too bitter.

*2 cups thinly sliced unpeeled baby zucchini, chilled*
*2 medium-size firm-ripe tomatoes, cored and thinly*
*    sliced*
*1 medium-size red onion, peeled, sliced paper thin,*
*    and separated into rings*
*³/₄ cup thinly sliced mushrooms (optional)*
*¹/₃ cup French Dressing*
*2 cups prepared mixed salad greens*

Mix all ingredients except greens, cover, and chill 1 hour, turning now and then. Line a salad bowl with the greens, mound zucchini mixture on top, and toss at the table (there should be enough dressing for the greens, too; if not add a little more).

NPS (4–6) (with mushrooms): 165–110 C, 0 mg CH, 60–40 mg S

VARIATION
**Okra Salad:** Prepare as directed but substitute baby okra for zucchini.

NPS (4–6) (with mushrooms): 170–115 C, 0 mg CH, 60–40 mg S

## WILTED CUCUMBERS

**4 servings**

> 2 medium-size cucumbers, peeled or not (as you
>     like) and sliced paper thin
> 1½ teaspoons salt
> 2 tablespoons boiling water
> 2 tablespoons sugar
> ⅓ cup white, tarragon, or cider vinegar
> Grinding of pepper

Layer cucumbers in a bowl, salting as you go, weight down, cover, and let stand at room temperature 1–2 hours. Drain, wash in a colander under cold running water, then drain and press out as much liquid as possible; pat dry on paper toweling. Mix water and sugar until sugar dissolves, add vinegar, pour over cucumbers, and toss well. Cover and chill 1–2 hours, mixing now and then. Top with a grinding of pepper and serve as is or in lettuce cups.

NPS: 45 C, 0 mg CH, 830 mg S

# RUSSIAN SALAD

**6 servings**

> 1 cup cold diced cooked potatoes
> 1 cup cold cooked cut green beans
> 1 cup cold diced cooked carrots
> 1 cup cold cooked green peas
> $^1/_3$ cup French Dressing
> $^1/_3$ cup mayonnaise
> 1 cup cold diced cooked beets
> 1 head Boston or romaine lettuce, trimmed and
>     chilled
> 1 tablespoon capers

Mix all vegetables except beets with French Dressing, cover, and chill 2–3 hours. Drain and save dressing; mix 1 tablespoon with mayonnaise, add to vegetables along with beets, and toss well. Mound on lettuce and top with capers.

NPS: 230 C, 5 mg CH, 190 mg S

# GREEN BEAN SALAD

**6 servings**

Cooked green beans in a spicy dressing.

> 1$^1/_2$ pounds green beans, boiled and drained, or 2
>     (8-ounce) packages frozen cut green beans,
>     cooked and drained by package directions
> 1 medium-size red onion, peeled and sliced thin

2 tablespoons minced fresh tarragon or $1/2$ teaspoon
    dried tarragon
1 clove garlic, peeled and crushed
2 teaspoons prepared spicy brown mustard
$1/2$ teaspoon salt
Pinch pepper
$1/2$ cup olive oil
3 tablespoons red or white wine vinegar

Place beans and onion in a large bowl. Blend together dressing ingredients, pour over beans and onion, and toss to mix. Cover and let stand at room temperature about 1 hour. Toss again and serve.

NPS: 205 C, 0 mg CH, 210 mg S

### DRIED BEAN SALAD

**4 servings**

2 cups any cold, well-drained, boiled dried beans
$1/3$ cup minced celery
$1/3$ cup minced sweet green pepper
$1/3$ cup minced yellow onion
3 tablespoons olive or other salad oil
2 tablespoons cider vinegar
$1/2$ teaspoon salt (about)
$1/8$ teaspoon pepper
2 tablespoons minced parsley

Mix all ingredients, cover, and chill several hours or overnight, tossing now and then. Taste for salt and adjust.

NPS: 215 C, 0 mg CH, 295 mg S

**Parmesan Bean Salad:** Prepare and chill salad as directed. Just before serving toss in ¼ cup finely grated Parmesan cheese.

NPS: 235 C, 5 mg CH, 390 mg S

**Bean and Beet Salad** (Makes 6 servings): Prepare as directed but add 1 (1-pound) can pickled beets, drained and diced, and 2 extra tablespoons olive oil.

NPS: 230 C, 0 mg CH, 415 mg S

## SALAD DRESSINGS

### FRENCH DRESSING (VINAIGRETTE)

**1 cup**

Called *vinaigrette* in France, French dressing is simply three to four parts olive oil to one part vinegar, seasoned with salt and pepper.

*¼ cup red or white wine vinegar*
*¼ teaspoon salt*
*⅛ teaspoon white pepper*
*¾ cup olive oil*

In a bowl mix vinegar, salt, and pepper with a wire whisk. Add oil and mix vigorously until well blended and slightly thickened. *(Note:* For a creamier dressing, beat over ice 1–2 minutes.) Use to dress green or vegetable salads. *(Note:* If you prefer, substitute any good salad oil for the olive oil and cider, malt, or other flavored vinegar for the wine vinegar.)

NP Tablespoon: 90 C, 0 mg CH, 35 mg S

**Garlic French Dressing:** Drop 1 peeled, bruised clove garlic into dressing and let stand 1–2 hours at room temperature; remove garlic before using dressing.

NP Tablespoon: 90 C, 0 mg CH, 35 mg S

**Tarragon French Dressing:** Make dressing with tarragon vinegar and add 1 tablespoon minced fresh or ½ teaspoon dried tarragon.

NP Tablespoon: 90 C, 0 mg CH, 35 mg S

**Roquefort French Dressing:** Prepare dressing as directed and crumble in 3 tablespoons Roquefort cheese. Cover and let stand several hours at room temperature before using.

NP Tablespoon: 95 C, 1 mg CH, 65 mg S

**Sweet French Dressing:** Prepare dressing as directed, then mix in ¼ cup each orange juice and honey or superfine sugar. Use to dress fruit salads.

NP Tablespoon (with honey): 105 C, 0 mg CH, 35 mg S
NP Tablespoon (with sugar): 105 C, 0 mg CH, 35 mg S

# FRESH HERB DRESSING

**³/₄ cup**

> *¹/₂ cup olive oil*
> *1 tablespoon minced fresh dill, tarragon, chervil, or*
> *fennel*
> *1 tablespoon minced chives*
> *¹/₄ teaspoon minced fresh marjoram (optional)*
> *¹/₂ teaspoon salt*
> *¹/₈ teaspoon pepper*
> *1 clove garlic, peeled and crushed (optional)*
> *¹/₄ cup tarragon vinegar*

Place oil, herbs, salt, pepper, and, if you like, the garlic in a shaker bottle or large glass measuring cup and let stand at room temperature 3–4 hours. Add vinegar and shake or stir well to blend. Use to dress any crisp green salad, using only enough to coat each leaf lightly. Save leftover dressing to use for other salads later (dressing will keep about 1 week).

NP Tablespoon: 80 C, 0 mg CH, 90 mg S

# BUTTERMILK DRESSING

**1¹/₂ cups**

Dieters, note just *how* low the calories are.

> *¹/₂ cup cider vinegar*
> *1 tablespoon salad oil*
> *1 teaspoon salt*

*¹/₈ teaspoon white pepper*
*1 cup buttermilk*

Shake all ingredients in a jar with a tight-fitting lid and use to dress cabbage or crisp green salads. *(Note:* Dressing will keep about a week in the refrigerator.)

NP Tablespoon: 10 C, 1 mg CH, 100 mg S

## LOW-CALORIE FRUIT DRESSING

**1¹/₃ cups**

> *1 clove garlic, peeled, bruised, and stuck on a toothpick*
> *5 tablespoons lemon juice*
> *1 cup pineapple, orange, or tangerine juice*
> *1 tablespoon light corn syrup or honey*
> *¹/₂ teaspoon salt*
> *¹/₄ teaspoon paprika*

Let garlic stand in lemon juice at room temperature 2 hours, then remove. Beat in remaining ingredients, cover, and chill. Shake well and use to dress fruit salads.

NP Tablespoon: 10 C, 0 mg CH, 55 mg S

## TANGY LOW-CALORIE SALAD DRESSING

**1½ cups**

Good with any green salad.

*1 tablespoon cornstarch*
*1 cup cold water*
*3 tablespoons salad oil*
*¼ cup cider vinegar*
*1 teaspoon salt*
*1 teaspoon sugar*
*2 tablespoons ketchup*
*1 teaspoon prepared mild yellow mustard*
*½ teaspoon paprika*
*½ teaspoon prepared horseradish*
*½ teaspoon Worcestershire sauce*
*½ teaspoon oregano*

Blend cornstarch and water and heat and stir over moderate heat until thickened and clear. Off heat, beat in remaining ingredients with a rotary beater or electric mixer. Cover and chill well. Shake before using.

NP Tablespoon: 20 C, 0 mg CH, 110 mg S

# MUSTARD SALAD DRESSING

**1½ cups**

2 tablespoons butter or margarine
2 tablespoons flour
1 cup milk
1 teaspoon salt
1½ teaspoons sugar
2 teaspoons powdered mustard blended with 2
    tablespoons cold water
⅓ cup cider vinegar

Melt butter in a small saucepan over moderately low heat, blend in flour, add milk slowly, and cook and stir until thickened and smooth. Mix in salt, sugar, and mustard paste. Add vinegar, 1 tablespoon at a time, beating well after each addition. Cool dressing, then cover and chill 2–3 hours. Beat well before using. Use to dress any cooked vegetable or seafood salad. *(Note:* Dressing keeps well about a week in refrigerator.)

NP Tablespoon (with butter): 20 C, 5 mg CH, 105 mg S

**VARIATION**
   **Extra-Low-Calorie Mustard Dressing:** Prepare as directed but use skim milk instead of regular.

NP Tablespoon (with butter): 15 C, 5 mg CH, 105 mg S

## DESSERTS

### HOT FRUIT COMPOTE

**6–8 servings**

A good basic recipe that can be varied a number of ways.

> *1 pound small ripe peaches or apricots, peeled, pitted, and halved*
> *1 pound small ripe pears, peeled, cored, and halved*
> *1 pound small ripe plums, peeled, pitted, and halved*
> *1 cup firmly packed light brown sugar*
> *$^1/_2$ cup orange juice mixed with $^1/_2$ cup water*
> *$^1/_4$ cup lemon juice*
> *1 tablespoon finely slivered orange rind*
> *2 tablespoons butter or margarine*

Preheat oven to 350° F. Arrange fruits in a large casserole. Combine sugar, orange juice mixture, lemon juice, and orange rind; pour over fruits, then dot with butter. Bake, uncovered, $^1/_2$ hour; serve hot.

NPS (6–8): 290–215 C, 10–5 mg CH, 50–40 mg S

**VARIATIONS**

**Spiced Hot Fruit Compote:** Add $^1/_2$ teaspoon cinnamon and $^1/_4$ teaspoon each ginger, nutmeg, and allspice to sugar mixture and proceed as directed.

NPS (6–8): 290–215 C, 10–5 mg CH, 50–40 mg S

**Brandied Hot Fruit Compote:** Prepare fruit compote as directed, using ½ cup each brandy and orange juice; also reduce lemon juice to 2 tablespoons.

NPS (6–8): 295–220 C, 10–5 mg CH, 50–40 mg S

**Curried Hot Fruit Compote:** First, heat and stir 1½ teaspoons curry powder in the butter called for in a flameproof casserole 1–2 minutes over moderate heat. Add fruits, substituting 2 cups pineapple chunks for the plums, pour in sugar mixture, mix well, and bake as directed. Serve hot with meat or poultry.

NPS (6–8): 290–215 C, 10–5 mg CH, 55–40 mg S

### FRIED APPLE RINGS

**6 servings**

Good as dessert or as a garnish for a roast pork platter.

*⅓ cup butter or margarine*
*4 medium-size cooking apples, cored but not peeled*
*    and sliced ½″ thick*
*Unsifted flour*

Heat butter in a large, heavy skillet over moderate heat 1 minute. Dredge apples in flour, shake off excess, and sauté, a few at a time, in butter about 10 minutes, turning often until lightly browned. Drain on paper toweling and serve hot.

NPS: 140 C, 20 mg CH, 80 mg S

**Curried Apple Rings:** Prepare as directed but sprinkle with 1–1½ teaspoons curry powder halfway through sautéing. *(Note:* Any of the following sautéed fruits may be curried the same way.)

NPS: 140 C, 20 mg CH, 80 mg S

**Sautéed Peaches or Apricots:** Pat 6 peach or apricot halves dry on paper toweling, then dredge and sauté 5–6 minutes as directed.

NPS: 130 C, 20 mg CH, 80 mg S

**Sautéed Halved Bananas:** Peel 6 underripe bananas and halve lengthwise. Dredge and sauté in butter about 5 minutes. Sprinkle lightly with salt and serve with meat or poultry.

NPS: 190 C, 20 mg CH, 80 mg S

### PORT WINE JELLY

**4–6 servings**

Both simple and sophisticated.

>  1⅓ *cups water*
>  2 *envelopes unflavored gelatin (3 envelopes if you*
>      *want to mold the jelly in a decorative mold)*
>  ⅔ *cup sugar*
>  *Juice of 1 lemon, strained through a fine sieve*
>  *Juice of 1 orange, strained through a fine sieve*
>  2 *cups dark ruby port wine*

Place water, gelatin, and sugar in a small saucepan, stir well to mix, then heat, stirring, over moderate heat about 5 minutes until sugar and gelatin are dissolved. Remove from heat and cool slightly. Mix in fruit juices and port. Pour into an ungreased 1-quart bowl or decorative mold, cover, and chill several hours until firm. To serve, spoon jelly into dessert glasses.

NPS (4–6): 315–210 C, 0 mg CH, 10–5 mg S

## LEMON OR LIME GRANITÉ

**1½ quarts (12 servings)**

Granité is a granular ice frozen without being stirred. It can be served at the mush stage or frozen hard, then scraped up in fine, feathery shavings. Particularly good topped with a little fruit liqueur or rum.

> *1 quart water*
> *2 cups sugar*
> *1 cup lemon or lime juice*
> *1 tablespoon finely grated lemon or lime rind*
> *Few drops yellow and/or green food coloring*

Bring water and sugar to a boil in a saucepan, stirring, then reduce heat and simmer, uncovered, 5 minutes. Cool, mix in juice and rind, and tint pale yellow or green. Pour into 3 refrigerator trays, cover, and freeze to a mush without stirring. Spoon into goblets and serve or freeze hard, scrape up with a spoon, and pile into goblets.

NPS (lemon): 135 C, 0 mg CH, 5 mg S

**Orange Granité:** Prepare as directed, substituting 1 quart orange juice for the water, reducing sugar to ³/₄ cup and lemon juice to 2 tablespoons; also use orange rind instead of lemon.

NPS: 85 C, 0 mg CH, 1 mg S

**Fruit Granité:** Boil 3 cups water and 1½ cups sugar into syrup as directed. Cool, add 2 tablespoons lemon juice and 2 cups puréed fruit (any berries, peaches, pineapple, sweet cherries); omit rind. Freeze and serve as directed.

NPS (with peach purée): 115 C, 0 mg CH, 5 mg S

**Coffee or Tea Granité:** Boil 1 cup each water and sugar into syrup as directed; cool, add 3 cups strong black coffee or tea and to tea mixture, add ¼ cup lemon juice. Freeze and serve as directed.

NPS (with coffee): 65 C, 0 mg CH, 1 mg S

**Melon Granité:** Mix 1 quart puréed ripe melon (any kind) with ½–1 cup sugar (depending on sweetness of melon) and 2 tablespoons lemon juice; let stand 1 hour at room temperature, stirring now and then, until sugar is dissolved. Freeze as directed.

NPS (½–1 cup sugar): 35–70 C, 0 mg CH, 1 mg S

# POACHED MERINGUE RING

6 servings

A beautiful base for sliced fresh berries or any dessert sauce.

*6 egg whites*
*⅛ teaspoon cream of tartar*
*¼ teaspoon salt*
*¾ cup superfine sugar*
*1 teaspoon vanilla*
*1 teaspoon lemon juice*
*¼ teaspoon almond extract*

Preheat oven to 325° F. Beat egg whites, cream of tartar, and salt with a rotary beater until foamy. Add sugar, a little at a time, beating well after each addition. Continue to beat until whites stand in stiff peaks. Fold in vanilla, lemon juice, and almond extract. Pack mixture in an ungreased 6-cup ring mold. Set mold in a shallow pan of cold water and bake, uncovered, 1 hour until meringue is lightly browned and pulls from the sides of mold. Remove meringue from oven and water bath and let cool upright in mold to room temperature. Loosen edges carefully with a spatula and unmold by inverting on a dessert platter. Cut into wedges and serve as is or with a generous ladling of dessert sauce (Algarve Apricot Sauce is especially good) or with sliced fresh berries.

NPS (without sauce or fruit): 115 C, 0 mg CH, 140 mg S

# MELBA SAUCE

**1½ cups**

Serve as a sauce for ice cream and fruit, or use to flavor milk shakes and sodas.

*1 pint fresh raspberries, washed, or 2 (10-ounce)*
    *packages frozen raspberries, thawed*
*⅓ cup red currant jelly*
*⅓–½ cup sugar*
*1 tablespoon cornstarch blended with 2*
    *tablespoons water*

Purée raspberries by buzzing 10–15 seconds in an electric blender at high speed or 5–10 seconds in a food processor fitted with the metal chopping blade; strain through a fine sieve. Pour into a saucepan, mix in jelly, sugar, and cornstarch paste, and cook and stir over moderate heat until thickened and clear. Cool, taste for sweetness, and add more sugar if needed.

NP Tablespoon: 30 C, 0 mg CH, 1 mg S

**VARIATIONS**
**Strawberry Sauce:** Prepare as directed, substituting 1 pint fresh strawberries or 2 (10-ounce) packages thawed frozen strawberries for the raspberries.

NP Tablespoon: 25 C, 0 mg CH, 1 mg S

**Currant Sauce:** Substitute 1 pint very ripe red or black currants for the raspberries and omit the currant jelly. If you like, mix the cornstarch with port wine or blackberry liqueur instead of water. Proceed as directed. Recipe too flexible for meaningful nutritional count.

## ALGARVE APRICOT SAUCE

**2¹/₄ cups**

In the south of Portugal lies the Algarve, where figs, peaches, and apricots grow. Women make them into a variety of sweets, among them this tart apricot sauce, luscious over a poached meringue.

> *1 (1-pound 14-ounce) can peeled whole apricots*
> *(do not drain)*
> *Juice and grated rind of 1 lemon*
> *1 cup firmly packed light brown sugar*
> *¹/₄ cup butter*

Pit apricots and purée in an electric blender at high speed or put through a food mill. Place in a small saucepan, add lemon juice, rind, and sugar, and simmer uncovered, stirring occasionally, 1 hour until thick and caramel colored. Remove from heat, stir in butter, and cool to room temperature. Serve over Poached Meringue Ring or as a dessert sauce for ice cream, sliced oranges or peaches.

NP Tablespoon: 50 C, 5 mg CH, 15 mg S

# LOW-CALORIE DESSERT TOPPING

**4 servings**

> 3 *tablespoons ice water*
> 3 *tablespoons nonfat dry milk powder*
> 2 *teaspoons lemon juice*
> *Few drops liquid noncaloric sweetener, 2 teaspoons low-calorie granulated sugar substitute, or 2 (1-gram) packets aspartame sweetener*
> 1/4 *teaspoon vanilla or almond extract*

Pour ice water into a chilled bowl, sprinkle powdered milk on surface, and beat with a rotary or electric beater until soft peaks form. Add lemon juice, sweeten to taste, add vanilla, and beat until stiff peaks form. Use at once.

NP Tablespoon: 15 C, 1 mg CH, 20 mg S

# Calorie Counter/Calories Burned per Hour

*H*ere is an unusual approach to personal fitness. The Calorie Counter is not a counter of calories consumed at each meal, but a counter of calories burned per hour at various weights.

This chart was developed to help you learn to balance your caloric intake (eating) with your caloric outgo (activity) as a healthful way of maintaining or losing weight.

For example, suppose you consume 2400 calories worth of food during a 24-hour period, and your level of activity is such that you burn off exactly 2400 calories as you work, sleep and play your way through the day. Supply and demand are equal. Your body neither calls on reserves to make up a deficit, nor does it deposit extra calories in the form of fat. You're maintaining your weight.

But, if you take in 2400 calories and burn off only 2300 calories of them, your body will "store" those 100 unnecessary calories in its fat cells until such time they're needed for energy.

One pound of fat is the equivalent of 3500 unnecessary calories. With this in mind, you can see that if you eat 100 calories more than you burn off through physical activity, at the end of 35 days you'll have gained a pound. And if you continue on at the same rate, you'll be 10 pounds heavier at the end of the year.

Most overweight problems are the result of being just a few calories per day out of balance. This chart shows you which kind of activities burn the most calories to assist you in getting your weight under control.

Many researchers are convinced that only through exercise can you properly control your weight without dangerously affecting the nutrients you need for healthful living. While it is true that you must burn 3500 calories to lose 1 pound of fat, you must remember that walking 20 minutes a day will burn up approximately 100 additional calories per day. In a year's time that is more than 10 pounds—pounds lost forever.

| ACTIVITY: | CALORIES BURNED PER HOUR: | | |
|---|---|---|---|
| | **99 pounds** | **125 pounds** | **152 pounds** |
| Badminton or Volleyball | 225 | 285 | 345 |
| Baseball | 185 | 234 | 284 |
| Basketball | 278 | 352 | 426 |
| Bicycling, on level, 5.5 mph | 198 | 251 | 304 |
| 13 mph | 424 | 537 | 651 |
| Bowling | 263 | 333 | 404 |
| Calisthenics | 198 | 251 | 304 |
| Dancing, moderate | 165 | 209 | 253 |
| Dressing or Showering | 126 | 160 | 193 |
| Driving | 118 | 150 | 181 |
| Eating | 55 | 70 | 85 |
| Gardening | 140 | 178 | 215 |
| Golf | 214 | 271 | 328 |
| Hill Climbing | 386 | 488 | 591 |
| Horseback Riding, trot | 267 | 338 | 409 |
| Housework | 161 | 203 | 246 |
| Mowing Grass | 176 | 222 | 269 |
| Office Work | 118 | 150 | 181 |
| Ping-Pong | 153 | 194 | 235 |
| Running, 7 mph | 552 | 699 | 847 |
| 9 mph | 757 | 959 | 1,161 |
| in place, 140 counts/ min. | 964 | 1,222 | 1,479 |
| Sailing | 118 | 150 | 181 |
| Shoveling Snow | 307 | 389 | 471 |
| Skating, moderate | 225 | 285 | 345 |
| Skiing, downhill | 382 | 483 | 585 |
| level, 5 mph | 463 | 586 | 709 |
| Sleeping | 46 | 59 | 71 |
| Swimming, crawl, 45 yd./min. | 345 | 437 | 529 |
| Tennis, moderate | 274 | 347 | 420 |
| vigorous | 386 | 488 | 591 |
| Walking, 2 mph | 139 | 176 | 213 |
| 4½ mph | 261 | 331 | 401 |
| Watching Television | 47 | 60 | 72 |
| Water Skiing | 307 | 391 | 473 |

# NOTES AND RECIPES

# NOTES AND RECIPES

# NOTES AND RECIPES

# NOTES AND RECIPES

# NOTES AND RECIPES

**Carol Tiffany** has been a food writer for more than twenty years. Her food and travel articles have appeared in *House Beautiful, Travel & Leisure, Cosmopolitan, Town & Country,* and *Early American Life;* in addition, she wrote a food column for the Recorder Publishing Company for fifteen years and a series on historic restaurants for *Antique Monthly.*

Carol has also been a food editor and recipe consultant at Western, Butterick, and Sterling Publishing companies. Although she continues to edit, the majority of her writing is now in fiction (where she finds her stories often focusing on food).